The
# Chester County Hospital
# Heart Book

## An Every Person's Guide

Verdi J. DiSesa, M.D.

The Chester County Hospital Heart Book:
*An Every Person's Guide*

Verdi J. DiSesa, M.D.
Chief, Cardiac Surgery
The CardioVascular Center
The Chester County Hospital
701 East Marshall Street
West Chester, Pennsylvania 19380
(610) 738-2690

Published by Windswept Productions
Felton, Pennsylvania 17322-0167
Copyright 2005
The Chester County Hospital Foundation and Verdi J. DiSesa, M.D.
ISBN Number 0-9764825-0-9
First Edition
Printed in the USA

EDITORS
Eleanor Boggs Shoemaker
Georg R. Sheets

ILLUSTRATOR
Jessica Huber

DESIGNER
Shade Tree Graphics

# TABLE OF CONTENTS

The philosophy of care at the CardioVascular Center at The Chester County Hospital is to engage individuals and families in the life-long management of cardiovascular disease. With that in mind, I wrote this book to inform and to engage. Management of your own cardiovascular health should be a process in which you participate actively.

Cardiovascular disease is our most important health problem (although today obesity, also a risk factor for heart disease, is giving it a run for its money). More people die of heart and blood vessel disease than of all forms of cancer combined. Many times more people suffer from cardiovascular disease than from car accidents or more publicized afflictions like AIDS. Cardiovascular disease is not something that most of us can ignore. However, we fear what we don't understand.

I hope that this book shines enough light into those dark spaces so that you feel empowered to engage in the preservation of your own heart health. With that intent, I have included in the appendix a prescription to get you started.

If you picked up this book, you're interested in the health of your heart and blood vessels. If you read it and "fill" the prescription offered, you will have begun to engage in a lifelong effort to protect and preserve the organ that the ancient medical philosophers considered the "seat of the soul."

*Verdi J. DiSesa, M.D.*

ACKNOWLEDGEMENTS

*With sincere thanks to my professional colleagues,
to special friends Wiggie and John Featherman,
Gretchen and Roy Jackson, Bonnie and Tom Musser,
and Diane and Bob Roskamp
whose contributions made this book possible,
and to H.L. Perry Pepper for his leadership and support
of The CardioVascular Center.*

♥

DEDICATION

*With love to*
*P.F.D., V.J.D. II, D.F.D., G.D.D. and A.H.D.*
*My own* sine qua non.

Dr. Verdi DiSesa was an invaluable advisor on health care when I ran for the Democratic Nomination for President in 2000. He was always clear and sensible. *The Chester County Hospital Heart Book: An Every Person's Guide* offers the same kind of advice. It serves as an excellent personal and family reference that provides understandable explanations about how the heart works, what can go wrong, and what treatment options are available.

Heart disease affects so many Americans, either directly or in our families and friends, that it is something that we must know more about. Reading Dr. DiSesa's book offers a pathway to better knowledge about the diagnosis and treatment of heart disease. With more information, it is possible to replace fear with awareness, and helplessness with a sense of involvement in and control of your own heart health.

I have learned many lessons as I have traveled across the country listening to citizens, seeking expert advice, and striving to address the real issues America has with health care. Among the most important of these lessons is the increasing need for individuals to be better informed about their own health and their own health care options. Then, they will be able to engage with doctors and other health professionals in the lifelong management of heart disease. Only by such engagement will we ensure a longer life with a healthier heart.

So, do what I myself have done and take advantage of the sound advice that Dr. DiSesa offers. His heart book is written for every person. My advice is that you read it.

*Bill Bradley*
*United States Senator (Ret.)*

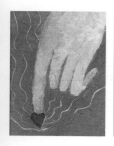

# Introduction

*Why a book about heart care?* Medical care of the heart and heart surgery, operations on the heart, are among the most important developments in modern medicine. The history of heart care is a history of the development of successful treatments for western society's most important health problem. More people die of cardiovascular disease, problems of the heart and the body's blood vessels, than from any other cause. In fact, more people die of this scourge than of cancer, AIDS, and other diseases which receive far more media attention.

Each year, three quarters of a million Americans suffer a heart attack in which the heart muscle is damaged. In about half of the victims, the damage to the heart is so severe that they die. That is almost one death per minute, 24 hours a day, 365 days a year.

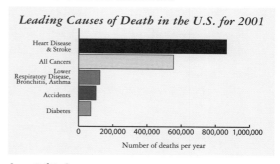

*Leading Causes of Death in the U.S. for 2001*

Heart disease is so prevalent that all our lives are touched by friends or relatives who have had a heart attack or heart surgery. Because of the advances in treatment of heart disease, many victims resume happy, productive lives. The modern medical successes in heart surgery have created the impression in some peoples' minds that heart disease is less a problem than, say, breast cancers in women. This is not even close to reality. Heart disease kills far more women than breast cancer does. But a recent survey of American women validated the fact that less than 10 percent knew that heart disease was the number one health problem in women.

If this book does no more than convince readers of the importance of heart disease awareness, it will have performed a valuable service. Knowledge of heart disease — prevention, treatment and cures — can help readers improve their own heart health and the heart health of the ones they love.

Improving heart health is what this book is really about. It also chronicles the state of a remarkable art and science that was developed from scratch in the second half of the twentieth century. In the late nineteenth century, distinguished professors of surgery in Europe, then the world capital of the surgical arts, concluded that little could be done to treat the heart with surgery, and all that could be done was already known. One distinguished surgeon, who even has abdominal surgical procedures named for him, concluded that any surgeon who dared operate on the heart should lose the respect of his colleagues.

This bold pronouncement was challenged briefly in the 1920s by courageous surgeons in Europe and the United States who tried to correct certain kinds of heart valve disease. There were sporadic successes, but often there were more failed operations than lives saved. It was not until World War II when the work of daring military surgeons matched surgical technology and innovative boldness to inaugurate the modern era of heart surgery.

Dr. Dwight Harken's work removing shrapnel from the hearts of wounded soldiers paved the way for his own and Dr. Charles Bailey's ultimately successful attempts to treat rheumatic heart disease of one of the heart valves. By modern standards, these operations were crude and imprecise. They were performed without modern knowledge about anesthesia and the care of the critically ill patient. The operations on valves inside the heart were performed with the heart still beating and supporting the circulation. At the time, there were no heart lung machines. Therefore, the surgeon could not stop the heart, open it and peer inside to see directly the disease and to verify the accuracy of the operation. Nonetheless, these pioneering operations did save and restore lives and constituted the dawn of modern heart surgery.

Harken and Bailey's efforts in the late 1940s were followed by an explosion of new technological developments led by surgeons such as Lillehei in Minnesota, Gibbon in Philadelphia, Kirklin in Minnesota and Alabama, and Shumway in Minnesota and Stanford. There were many others. It is instructive to note that all of these developments remain fairly recent. The first heart-lung machines were developed in the 1950s. The first heart valve prostheses to replace diseased valves were developed in the early 1960s. The first heart transplant was done in 1967 and the first modern coronary bypass operation was not performed until 1968. No artificial heart kept any human alive longer than one day — until 1980 — and modern valve repair operations were not widely applied until even later.

So, modern heart surgery is a relatively recent success story. Heart operations are now among the most frequently performed major surgical procedures. Modern heart surgery has been the most studied and scrutinized field of human endeavor, let alone medical procedures. Many studies assessing the efficacy and cost of heart operations have been undertaken, some by surgeons, various foundations and agencies interested in the quality of medical care, state governments, and the federal government, in its role as administrator of the Medicare health care system. For these reasons an informed public needs to know about these medical procedures. This book aims to serve that purpose.

Modern heart surgery is not brain surgery. It's just as challenging, but more important, since heart disease is a more prevalent health problem than diseases that require operations on the brain. Welcome to the adventure in healing that modern heart care offers. There are wonderful ways to help people with today's cardiac surgical tools. There remains much to learn. Following is a summary of what has been accomplished in heart care, what can be done today with operations designed to heal damaged hearts, and what may lie in the future. ♥

# Human Vascular Anatomy

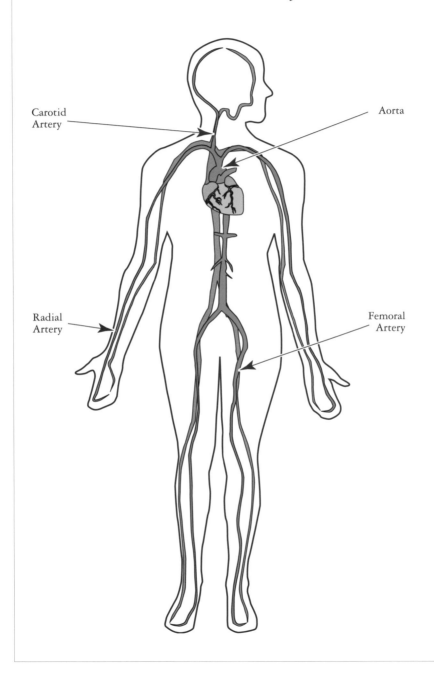

Carotid
Artery

Aorta

Radial
Artery

Femoral
Artery

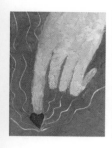

# CHAPTER 1

# Basic Heart Anatomy and Physiology

*The heart is a muscular pump* that sits slightly to the left of the middle of the chest directly behind the sternum (breastbone). Literally, it is the "heart" of the circulatory system that delivers blood and oxygen throughout the body tissues. Blood lacking oxygen is re-collected in the heart, which then delivers it to the lungs where oxygen is restored. (See illustration, opposite.)

The heart is actually two pumps, each operating in parallel with the other. The right heart collects the unoxygenated blood from all the body's veins and pumps it to the lungs. The oxygenated blood returns from the lungs to the left side of the heart, which then pumps it to the body. (See illustration on next page.) The cycle continues indefinitely: oxygenated blood pumped by the left heart to the body; unoxygenated blood collected in the right heart where oxygen is re-charged, oxygenated blood returned to the left heart for delivery to the tissues. In a normal size adult at rest, the heart beats about 75 times a minute. The heartbeat can be felt by taking your pulse in the neck, wrist, or groin. The pumping action of the heart, the circulation of blood, proceeds at a rate of about five liters per minute, approximately the equivalent of a bit more than a gallon a minute. With exertion, the output of the heart can double or triple. In highly trained athletes, cardiac outputs as high as 50 liters per minute have been recorded.

Both the right and the left sides of the heart are made up of two chambers. The atrium is an antechamber in which blood returning from the body (right atrium) or the lungs (left atrium) is collected. The actual pumping chambers are the right ventricle,

## Internal Heart Anatomy

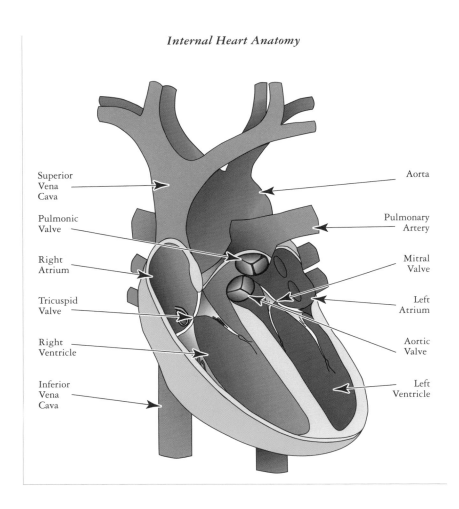

Superior Vena Cava

Aorta

Pulmonic Valve

Pulmonary Artery

Right Atrium

Mitral Valve

Tricuspid Valve

Left Atrium

Right Ventricle

Aortic Valve

Inferior Vena Cava

Left Ventricle

which pushes blood to the lungs, and the left ventricle, which delivers it to the rest of the body. Normal electrical signals in the heart cause the atria to contract first, completing filling of the ventricles — which then contract, expelling the blood from the heart.

The heart has valves, which are flaps of thin, veil-like tissue ensuring that blood only flows forward in the heart. There are two valves on each side of the heart. One set of valves, the atrio-ventricular valves, is at the junction between the atrium and the ventricle on each side of the heart. The tricuspid valve prevents the flow of blood backward into the right atrium when the right ventricle contracts.

The mitral valve does the same job on the left side of the heart, preventing back flow of blood into the left atrium when the left ventricle contracts. There are also valves at the outlets to the right and the left ventricles that prevent backflow of blood into the ventricles when they are relaxed. The pulmonic valve does this job for the right ventricle. The aortic valve does the same job for the left ventricle.

Blood is carried throughout the body by blood vessels, which are cylindrical tubes with a wall and a hollow center. The two primary types of blood vessels are arteries and veins. Arteries take blood away ("a" for "artery" and for "away") from the heart. Veins return blood to it. Blood returns to the right heart through the superior (from the head and arms) and inferior (from the lower body) venae cavae and to the left heart via the pulmonary ("pulmonary" means having to do with the lungs) veins. The right heart pumps blood to the lungs through the pulmonary artery. The left heart puts it into the aorta.

The aorta is an important structure since the entire blood supply to the body passes through it. It can have diseases of its own. The aorta has segments in the chest (the thoracic aorta) and in the abdomen (the abdominal aorta). At about the level of the umbilicus (navel), the aorta

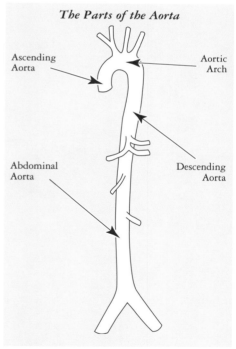

**The Parts of the Aorta**

Ascending Aorta

Aortic Arch

Abdominal Aorta

Descending Aorta

divides into two branches that supply blood to the pelvis and the legs.

When the aorta first exits the heart, blood in it passes upward in the chest. For this reason, the first segment of the aorta is called the ascending aorta. The first branches off the aorta are the right and left coronary arteries, which come off just above the aortic valve.

These arteries supply blood that keeps the heart muscle alive. Near the top of the chest, the aorta makes a curve and then turns downward. The horizontal part of that curve is called the aortic arch. All of the blood supply of the head and arms is derived from three major branches in the arch of the aorta. After the aorta makes the turn downward, it descends towards the diaphragm that marks the boundary between the chest and the abdomen. This part of the aorta is called the descending thoracic aorta.

Most diseases of the heart and blood vessels that afflict adults affect the aortic and mitral valves on the left side of the heart, the aorta and its branches, and the coronary arteries that supply blood to the heart. Disease of the coronary arteries can cause heart attacks and

### The Coronary Arteries

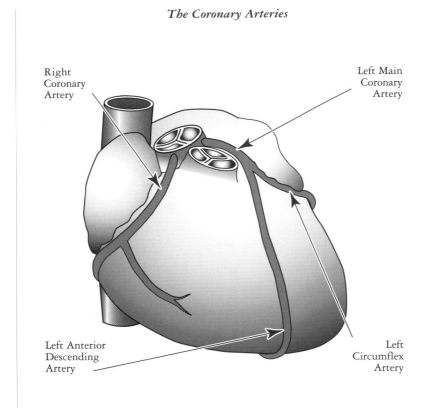

Right Coronary Artery

Left Main Coronary Artery

Left Anterior Descending Artery

Left Circumflex Artery

death, and therefore, it is important to have a more detailed understanding of the anatomy of the coronary arteries.

The right and the left coronary arteries supply different regions of the heart muscle but the areas that they supply are not rigidly restricted to the right or the left hearts. In fact, both vessels can supply blood to both sides of the heart. The right coronary artery supplies the majority of blood to the right ventricle, and then, in about 85 percent of people, continues to supply the underside, or diaphragmatic, portion of the heart. In 15 percent of people, a branch of the left coronary artery supplies this part of the heart. The left coronary artery supplies most of the blood to the left ventricle. Since the left ventricle is the more common site of heart attacks, in some senses, the left coronary artery is the most important vessel supplying blood to the heart.

The left coronary artery has a short segment called the "left main" which is about one-inch long. The left main coronary branches into the left anterior descending (LAD) coronary and the left circumflex (LCx) coronary arteries. The LAD provides blood to the anterior surface of the heart, and is the artery that supplies the largest proportion of blood to the heart in most people. The LCx supplies the lateral wall, or side, of the heart. As noted, in 15 percent of people, it contributes a branch that supplies the bottom of the heart near the diaphragm.

Diseases in these key cardiac or aortic structures are what cause death and disability from cardiovascular disease. Obstructions in the coronary arteries can cause reductions in blood supply to the heart muscle. When the supply of blood through these obstructed vessels is inadequate to meet the heart's needs for blood and oxygen, damage to the heart muscle — heart attacks — can occur. The heart valves, particularly the mitral and aortic valves, can develop diseases that cause leakage or scarring and narrowing of the valve. These conditions affect the flow of blood through the heart and can increase the workload and decrease the effectiveness of the contraction, the squeezing force, of each beat of the heart. The aorta and its branches can develop diseases, which cause weakening and enlargement of blood vessels. These enlargements are called aneurysms and can cause problems if they push on other structures. The most catastrophic problem associated with aneurysms is acute rupture, which can be fatal rapidly. Another important disease of the thoracic aorta is called aortic dissection. In this condition, the blood inside the vessel gets into the wall of the artery through a tear in its inner lining. The pumping of the blood causes dissection, or movement, of this blood forward or backward inside the wall of the vessel. This dissection of blood inside the wall of the aorta can cause serious problems.

This chapter has presented enough of the anatomy and physiology (biological functioning) of the heart and the blood vessels to permit the reader to develop an appreciation for the nature of diseases of the heart and blood vessels. This knowledge is also important for understanding how diseases of the heart and blood vessels are diagnosed and treated. ♥

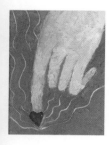

# CHAPTER 2

# Coronary Artery Disease

*The coronary arteries* supply blood to the heart muscle. Disease in these vessels can cause heart attack and other problems. This is the disease that is America's most important public health problem and from which more people die than any other cause. Therefore, an understanding of the basics of coronary artery disease (CAD) is important for anyone interested in improving his or her own heart health, the heart health of a loved one, or the heart health of mankind in general.

Atherosclerosis, sometimes called "hardening" of the arteries, is the most frequent and the most common cause of coronary artery disease. There are inflammatory (inflammation is the body's response to injury) processes and some congenital defects that can affect the coronary arteries, but CAD from atherosclerosis is the most important. Atherosclerosis causes problems as a result of the narrowings of

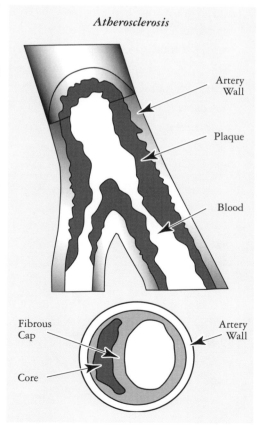

*Atherosclerosis*

Artery Wall

Plaque

Blood

Fibrous Cap

Core

Artery Wall

the coronary arteries. The narrowings restrict the flow of blood to the heart muscle and cause symptoms, heart attack, and death.

Atherosclerosis is the build-up of fatty deposits (atheromas) in the wall of the coronary artery (or any artery in the body for that matter). These fatty deposits build up gradually with time and may not produce any noticeable clinical effect until they produce at least a 60 percent to 70 percent reduction in the orifice of the blood vessel. There are many known risk factors for the development of coronary atherosclerosis, but the exact cause of this process and why it affects some people more than others, why some vessels are affected and others are not, continue to remain largely unknown. Risk factors for CAD will be discussed in the next chapter.

As a living biologic organ the heart has a need for blood and oxygen, even at rest. The heart's need for oxygen increases with increasing physical or mental/emotional activity. The coronary arteries supply blood to the heart to meet these demands. When the flow of blood in the coronary arteries is restricted by atherosclerosis, the heart's demand for blood and oxygen may exceed the coronary arteries' capacity to supply it. Under these circumstances, the patient may experience symptoms. When the imbalance between supply and demand is severe and prolonged enough, damage to the heart muscle, a heart attack, may occur.

The classic symptom of inadequate blood supply to the heart muscle is a chest discomfort syndrome commonly called angina pectoris. While angina is often referred to as chest "pain," many patients will deny pain and report a discomfort more like a pressure or a squeezing sensation. This can be quite severe. Angina can be brought on by increasing activity or emotional distress ("demand" angina), and usually subsides with rest. Some patients put a small pill called nitroglycerine under the tongue (which is rapidly absorbed into the system). This drug causes relaxation of blood vessels, reducing the work of the heart and often leading to more rapid relief of symptoms.

Some patients with more severe narrowings get angina at rest ("supply" angina). In these cases, the supply of blood to the heart is limited by the coronary obstructions and even minor changes in the heart's demand for oxygen can cause symptoms. Some patients lack a warning system of any kind and have never experienced angina, even though they may have significant CAD. This condition is sometimes most notable in patients with diabetes who do have risk factors for CAD but do not get symptoms like typical angina.

Angina, when it occurs, can be associated with other symptoms like sweatiness, nausea, shortness of breath, or neck, jaw, back, arm, or hand pain. Some patients have very atypical symptoms that appear to be completely unrelated to the heart. The most common of these are indigestion or burping. Such atypical presentations are particularly common in women. Until recently, the importance of CAD in women was under-appreciated and often less aggressively investigated and treated. Because of the many manifestations that angina may take in all patients, often a patient's first reaction is to think that it is something else. It has been said that "denial" is the first symptom of heart disease. It must not be, however, since prompt diagnosis and treatment can be life saving.

### Normal EKG

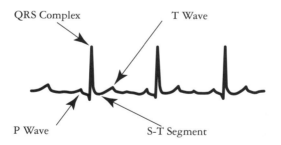

QRS Complex

T Wave

P Wave

S-T Segment

Angina pectoris can be associated with typical changes on the electrocardiogram, or EKG. This test measures the changes in the electrical activity in real time and results are obtained by placing "leads," or wires attached to the EKG machine, in contact with the arms and legs and over the chest. Inadequate blood supply to the heart muscle produces characteristic changes in the EKG tracing when the heart is not getting enough blood. Since multiple leads of the EKG are examined, the leads with the changes provide clues to the location of the heart attack. When the balance between the heart's demand for blood and the supply from the coronary arteries is restored, the EKG returns to its normal baseline state as, or after, the symptoms of angina subside.

More prolonged angina with persistent disparity between the heart's need for blood and its supply can produce irreversible damage to the heart muscle. This is called a heart attack. A portion of the heart muscle dies and is replaced in time by scar. When this area is large enough, permanent damage may be done to the function of the heart. This can lead to heart failure, or even death, immediately, or later. Acute damage to the heart can also cause potentially fatal abnormal heart rhythms. This is one reason why intensive care monitoring, which has been shown to reduce mortality from heart attack, is so important early after the event.

The mechanism of disease producing heart attacks is apparently different from the way angina is produced. In angina, a fixed narrowing leads to inadequate blood flow to the heart usually under situations of increased demand. Heart attacks, it is now believed, occur when a coronary artery plaque ruptures and leads to sudden total closure of the coronary artery. This plaque may not have produced a significant narrowing prior to the rupture event. Plaques that are prone to rupture apparently have weaker coverings or caps that can be knocked off by the force of flowing blood. (See illustration.) Removing the cap of such a "vulnerable" plaque exposes the material in the plaque to platelets, small blood cells that produce clots, and blood proteins, which lead to blood clotting. The exposed plaque material causes platelets to stick. Platelets attract a protein mesh, which forms a clot that completely blocks the flow of blood to the heart muscle beyond the plaque. When prolonged several hours, this interruption of blood flow causes irreversible heart muscle damage.

Such a heart attack that affects the entire thickness of the wall of the heart in the area affected can produce what is called a "transmural" myocardial infarction (heart attack). This pattern of

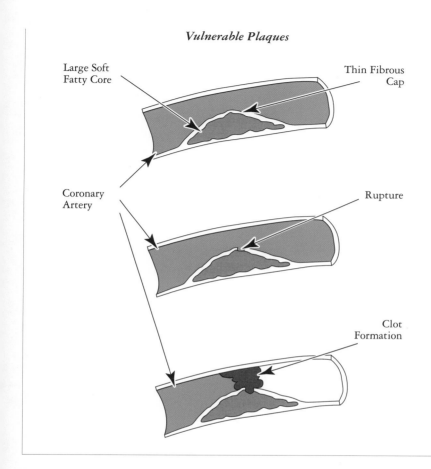

**Vulnerable Plaques**

Large Soft
Fatty Core

Thin Fibrous
Cap

Coronary
Artery

Rupture

Clot
Formation

injury is associated with typical EKG changes that involve elevation of a portion of the EKG called the "S-T segment." Such S-T segment elevation infarctions are thought to occur consistently in the manner described above. The importance of this will be clear when we discuss the treatment of coronary artery disease.

Between reversible angina and S-T segment elevation

**EKG Changes Due to
Myocardial Infarction
(Heart Attack)**

S-T Segment
Elevation

infarctions is a spectrum of conditions known as intermediate coronary syndromes. These are not typically associated with S-T segment elevations, but some degree of non-transmural heart muscle injury can occur. One entity in the spectrum of acute coronary syndromes, therefore, is called a non-S-T segment elevation infarction.

Acute coronary syndromes are thought to be associated with unstable coronary artery plaques but not the sudden complete obstruction that leads to an S-T segment elevation infarction. The blood platelets appear to have an important role in the unstable plaque activity associated with acute coronary syndromes. Therefore, as we will discuss, drugs that inhibit platelet stickiness appear to play an important role in the management of patients with these conditions between angina and heart attack. ♥

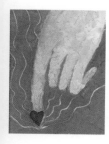

CHAPTER 3

# Fats and Other Risk Factors

*While the exact causes* of coronary artery disease and atherosclerosis are not understood, a number of risk factors have been
identified, many of which can be controlled, or at least modified, to
lessen the threat of disease. Risk factor identification and modification are the components of a program to try to prevent cardiovascular
disease. While this book is mainly about the wonderful advances in
diagnosis and treatment of heart disease, the book's ultimate goal is
to help prevent heart disease occurrence in the first place.

Abnormalities of cholesterol and other fats, collectively called
lipids, are among the most prevalent and widely recognized risk
factors for cardiovascular disease. The standard used to be to try to
keep the total cholesterol level in the blood less than 200, plus your
age (the units of cholesterol measurement are mg/100 ml). More
recent standards suggest that a total cholesterol less than 200 mg/
100 ml is desirable.

More important than the absolute value of the cholesterol level
are the levels of components of total cholesterol, namely low-density
lipoproteins (LDL) and high-density lipoproteins (HDL). A lipopro-
tein is simply a fat attached to a protein. The cholesterol in blood is
part of a group of lipoproteins. Again, the ratio between these
lipoproteins is as important as their levels. Higher LDL is associated
with increased risk of cardiovascular disease — higher HDL with
reduced risk. The lower the ratio of LDL to HDL, the lower the
cardiovascular risk. The goal is to try to get the LDL under 100
mg/100ml and as close to 70 mg/100 ml, as possible, and the HDL
at least 45 mg/100 ml or higher.  These yield a desirable LDL:HDL

ratio of less than 2:1.

A number of factors can modify the levels of cholesterol and the ratio between its various forms in the blood. A diet high in saturated fats has adverse effects on total cholesterol and the ratio of its components. High fat diets are also high calorie diets. Excess weight, obviously related to excess caloric intake, also can raise total cholesterol and LDL. Conversely, exercise, which burns calories, can lower weight and thereby have a beneficial effect on cholesterol and LDL. Exercise also has the benefit of leading to increases in HDL, so it has a double beneficial effect on the LDL:HDL ratio.

Smoking is bad for you. Not only are there elements in tobacco smoke that can cause emphysema and cancer of the lung and other parts of the airways, nicotine is damaging to blood vessels. Nicotine causes constriction of the muscles in the walls of blood vessels and can have deleterious effects on the linings of blood vessels as well. Cigarette smoke also reduces HDL levels.

Patients with diabetes (high blood sugar) are at increased risk of developing cardiovascular disease, especially because they can have disease in smaller blood vessels which are harder to treat. Diabetes comes in two types, Type I, or insulin-dependent diabetes, and Type II, or non-insulin-dependent diabetes. Type I used to be called juvenile-onset diabetes, and Type II was known as adult-onset diabetes. While it is true that virtually all children who develop diabetes are insulin-dependent, this stratification based on age of onset has proven to be less useful.

The effects of diabetes on blood vessels can be modulated. Tight control of blood sugar to keep it close to normal (about 100 mg/100 ml) is important. Success at regulation of blood sugar in this way can be measured by checking a blood test called Hemoglobin A1C. This test reflects how well blood sugar has been controlled over time.

Most adults with Type II diabetes are overweight (conversely, most children with Type I diabetes are thin). Weight loss facilitates maintenance of more normal blood sugar and may eliminate the need for insulin or other medications to control blood sugar levels.

In addition, weight loss has the other additional benefits of reducing unfavorable cholesterol levels.

Obesity, by itself, is a risk factor for the development of cardiovascular disease. Unfortunately, obesity, now often thought of as part of the metabolic syndrome, is epidemic in our society, and alarmingly so among young people. In fact, childhood obesity is becoming an epidemic in the United States and looms as a major public health problem. Overweight people can have problems with blood sugar, as noted, but also with high blood pressure and inactivity. An inactive life-style contributes to over-eating, and thus to obesity, and denies the person the positive health benefits of exercise.

High blood pressure (hypertension) is also a risk factor for cardiovascular disease. In the early phases, hypertension is completely asymptomatic. It exerts its harmful effects on the heart, blood vessels, the kidney, and the brain slowly over time. The only way hypertension can be detected early is to measure the blood pressure regularly. Blood pressure is measured by two numbers: the systolic pressure, which is the blood pressure when the heart is contracting, and the diastolic pressure, which is the blood pressure between beats when the heart is relaxed.

A normal blood pressure is 120/80 mmHg (millimeters of Mercury, the standard units for measuring blood pressure). To reduce the risk of heart disease, it is desirable to keep the systolic pressure at 130 or less and the diastolic pressure at 90 or less. This can be accomplished with a variety of medications. In many patients, these medications are necessary for controlling blood pressure. In some patients, the amount of such medicines can be reduced or possibly eliminated by a program of diet, exercise, and weight loss.

A diet with limited salt and reduced calories may have a beneficial effect on blood pressure. Salt restriction seems to be important in treating this disease whose cause is often not detectable. Similarly, excess weight can contribute to elevated blood pressure. Excess weight can be a cause or a result of a sedentary life-style. A program of exercise can have a beneficial effect, not just on well-being, weight, and cholesterol, but also on blood pressure. Attention to hypertension, at times called the "silent killer" since symptoms don't occur early, is an important component of heart health.

Modern thinking about risk factors for heart disease has led to development of the concept of the metabolic syndrome. The metabolic syndrome incorporates obesity as a risk factor, but includes a constellation of other conditions that increase the risk of heart disease. Central obesity (excessive fat tissue in and around the abdomen) is the defining characteristic. The others are abnormalities of blood fats, raised blood pressure, resistance to the action of the hormone, insulin, which normally controls blood sugar, a prothrombotic state in which there is an increased tendency for the blood to clot, and a condition of increased inflammation in the entire body system. All of these are risk factors for heart attack and other forms of cardiovascular disease.

Popularly, stress has been considered a risk factor for cardiovascular disease. Certain hormones that circulate in the blood when a person is under emotional or physical stress may contribute directly to heart disease. Probably the more important effect of stress on heart disease is indirect. A stressful life may be associated with reduced exercise, over-eating and excess weight, smoking, and high blood pressure. All of these are known factors that increase the risk of blood vessel disease. Stress reduction may lower risk of heart disease by reducing these clearly identified associated risk factors.

The above are all risk factors that we should identify and modify to reduce the risk of heart disease. Clearly, however, understanding of all the factors that produce cardiovascular disease is incomplete. While there are genetic tendencies to abnormal cholesterol levels, high blood pressure, and diabetes, there are other genetic factors important in the development of cardiovascular disease that have not yet been identified. Therefore, one of the strongest predictors of risk of cardiovascular disease is a family history. This is a particularly powerful risk factor when there is a history of premature atherosclerosis, that is blood vessel disease occurring at a relatively young age (in the thirties or forties).

Someday, perhaps relatively soon, it may be possible to identify precisely what the genes controlling these risks are. It may even be possible someday to repair defective genes that predispose an individual to cardiovascular disease. Today we must recognize that a family history containing close relatives with cardiovascular disease is a powerful risk for cardiovascular disease in others from that family group. When an individual has such a history, it provides even more motivation to search for and correct as many modifiable risk factors as possible.

The main goal of preventive cardiology, since heart disease is so prevalent in our society, is to identify our risk factors for heart and blood vessel disease. Beyond identification, modification of diet and life style are essential to reduce risk factors. Sometimes this will also require the use of medications. The best treatment for heart disease is to prevent it.

Following a program aimed at preventing this disease can have a significant impact on cardiovascular health. ♥

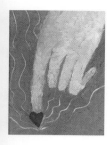

# CHAPTER 4

# Valvular Heart Disease

*In adults,* nearly all valvular heart disease is acquired, and less often the result of a congenital heart defect. The valves most commonly affected are those on the left side of the heart, namely the aortic and mitral valves. (See illustration.) Abnormalities of these valves can be quite severe even before significant symptoms develop. This is because the heart has a wonderful capability of adapting to abnormal loads of pressure and volume before it starts to fail and produce functional abnormalities and symptoms.

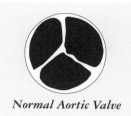

*Normal Aortic Valve*

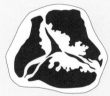

*Valve with Aortic Stenosis*

The two abnormalities that the aortic and mitral valves can develop are narrowing, called stenosis; and leaking, called insufficiency, or sometimes regurgitation. Sometimes valves develop both stenosis and insufficiency since the process that distorts the valve by narrowing it can also render the valve incompetent. Valves can become narrowed as the result of either degenerative or inflammatory conditions. Degenerative aortic stenosis is the most common valve abnormality in adults. In this condition, the leaflets of the aortic valve become scarred and stiffened, narrowing the orifice of the valve and increasing the pressure that the heart must generate to push the blood past the valve. As this scarring progresses, deposits of calcium, which can be quite large, contribute to the stiffening of the leaflets and the narrowing of the valve. The precise cause of this problem is not known, but it seems, in part, to be a product of aging. Most patients who develop this condition are in the eighth and ninth decades of life. There is some recent evidence that abnormalities of lipoproteins may contribute to the development of aortic stenosis. This could be a risk factor for the disease that is modifiable by medications or other methods.

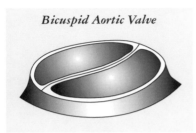

*Bicuspid Aortic Valve*

Some people are born with an aortic valve with two, rather than the normal three, leaflets. (See illustration.) These valves function normally for forty or fifty years. Eventually, probably because the flow of blood past a two-leaflet valve is somewhat turbulent, these valves can scar, stiffen, and calcify. These patients can develop symptomatic aortic stenosis at a younger age than those with classic degenerative valve disease.

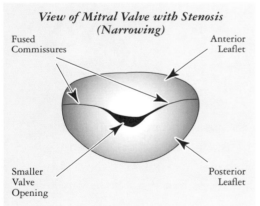

*View of Mitral Valve with Stenosis (Narrowing)*

Fused Commissures

Anterior Leaflet

Smaller Valve Opening

Posterior Leaflet

The mitral valve can also develop stenosis. The most common condition that leads to mitral stenosis is rheumatic heart disease. This disease is caused by a streptococcus bacterium that causes inflammation of the heart and valves, especially the mitral valve. This is acute rheumatic fever. Rheumatic fever typically occurs in young patients; many adults do not recall having it — or it was never discovered that they had suffered from this acute condition. Although the inflammation subsides, in time the mitral valve can develop scarring, calcification, and narrowing. The valve can become scarred, furthermore, in such a way that it also leaks. Typically, this process occurs slowly. Most patients with rheumatic mitral stenosis develop symptoms in their forties, fifties or sixties. Today, there are antibiotics that can cure streptococcal infections.

These have reduced but not eliminated rheumatic heart disease, however, since patients in developing countries, or even disadvantaged people in developed countries, do not always have access to medical services to diagnose and treat acute rheumatic fever. This population, therefore, is still at risk for developing chronic rheumatic heart disease, the most common manifestation of which is mitral stenosis.

Degenerative mitral insufficiency is the valve abnormality second in frequency to aortic stenosis. This abnormality is caused by degeneration, some of which may be genetically determined, of the structures of the mitral valve. The mitral valve has not only the valve leaflets, but is supported by an annulus (ring) that attaches the leaflet to the heart at the junction of the atrium and ventricles. In addition, the mitral valve leaflets are attached to specialized areas of the left ventricle, called papillary muscles, by thin strings called chordae tendineae. This entire apparatus must be functional for the mitral valve to be competent.

*The Mitral Valve Apparatus*

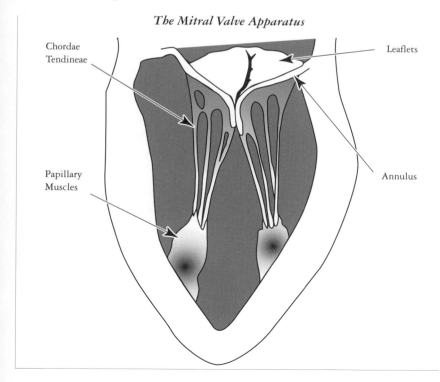

Chordae Tendineae

Leaflets

Papillary Muscles

Annulus

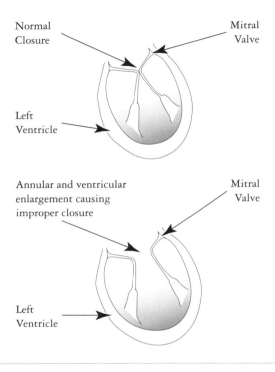

*Changes in Heart Size and Shape
Affect the Function of the Mitral Valve*

Normal
Closure

Mitral
Valve

Left
Ventricle

Annular and ventricular
enlargement causing
improper closure

Mitral
Valve

Left
Ventricle

Sometimes enlargement of the heart from some other cause is sufficient to cause leakage of the mitral valve. As the heart, particularly the left ventricle, enlarges, it stretches the mitral annulus. When the annulus enlarges enough, the increased distance between the valve leaflets can prevent their coming together to close properly when the ventricle squeezes. This can lead to leakage of the valve. Part of the blood ejected from the left ventricle goes backward into the left atrium and does not contribute to supplying blood and oxygen to the body. To compensate, the body holds on to fluid (so that there is more to pump forward with every heartbeat). This enlarges the heart even more. Ironically, this stretches the mitral annulus further, increasing the valve insufficiency and perpetuating the downward spiraling process.

Mitral insufficiency can be caused also when the chordae stretch or break or when there is enlargement and redundancy of the mitral leaflets. The cause of these tissue changes is not completely understood, but there almost certainly is a genetic component. Stretched or broken chords or enlarged leaflets can prolapse backward into the left atrium every time the heart beats. This can occur without valve leakage and has been called the "mitral valve prolapse" syndrome. When prolapse is severe enough, significant valve leakage can occur.

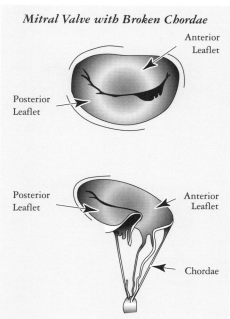

*Mitral Valve with Broken Chordae*

Anterior Leaflet

Posterior Leaflet

Posterior Leaflet

Anterior Leaflet

Chordae

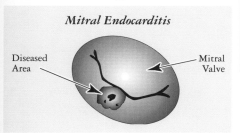

*Mitral Endocarditis*

Diseased Area

Mitral Valve

Infection of any of the heart valves, a condition called endocarditis, can cause valve insufficiency. A virulent enough infection can lead to inflammation, damage, and destruction of the mitral valve leaflets, annulus, and/or chordae. When this destruction is severe, significant valve leakage can occur. Endocarditis can also affect the aortic valve. By a similar destructive mechanism, endocarditis of the aortic valve leaflets may disrupt their integrity, or the integrity of the leaflet attachments to the aortic valve annulus, producing severe leakage of the aortic valve.

Other degenerative conditions of the aortic valve leaflet tissue can lead to aortic insufficiency. As with degenerative mitral valve disease, there is probably a genetic component. In these cases, one or more aortic valve leaflets may become redundant and prolapsing. This causes failure of valve leaflet apposition and leads to significant leakage of blood back into the ventricle when it is relaxed.

Stenosis or insufficiency of the pulmonic valve is extremely rare in adult patients. The most common reason for an adult patient to have a pulmonic valve abnormality is as a residual of a congenital condition, which was probably treated when the person was a child.

Abnormalities of the tricuspid valve are the other conditions seen most commonly in adults. Rheumatic fever may affect the tricuspid valve, directly producing tricuspid stenosis or, more commonly, insufficiency in a manner analogous to the way in which this disease affects the mitral valve. The tricuspid valve may also develop functional insufficiency — that is, leakage due to enlargement of the valve and surrounding structures, and not to an intrinsic valve defect. As a consequence of mitral stenosis or insufficiency, patients may develop elevated blood pressure in the pulmonary veins. This is transmitted to the lungs and backwards to the right ventricle. As the right ventricle responds to this increased pressure and sometimes volume load, it may enlarge. As it does so, the tricuspid valve annulus may also enlarge leading to tricuspid insufficiency.

A similar mechanism may lead to tricuspid insufficiency in other conditions, which enlarge the heart. Heart failure from any cause may produce enough cardiac enlargement to stretch the tricuspid valve so that it leaks. Lung conditions may do so also by increasing the pressure the right ventricle must generate to pump blood to the lungs. Just as in mitral stenosis, this extra pressure can lead to right heart enlargement and tricuspid insufficiency. Finally, endocarditis can affect the tricuspid valve. When destruction of the tricuspid valve apparatus, which like the mitral valve includes annulus, leaflets, and chordae, is severe, significant tricuspid insufficiency may occur.

Heart valve disease may affect one valve or several heart valves simultaneously. The same condition may produce abnormalities of more than one valve. Alternatively, as described, one valve abnormality may produce abnormal loads on the heart that cause other valve abnormalities. For example, aortic stenosis can cause enough increased load on the heart to produce mitral insufficiency. Both abnormalities can get better when the aortic valve condition is fixed.

Although several different valve abnormalities may exist singly or in combination, the spectrum of symptoms produced by valvular heart disease is relatively limited. Patients who become symptomatic may have fatigue, shortness of breath, chest discomfort, dizziness or fainting, or fluid retention. Some may have a combination of these symptoms. Some may have all of them.

In general, fatigue is caused by inadequate delivery of blood to the tissues of the body. It is easy to imagine that both aortic and mitral stenosis may cause this symptom since both problems make it harder for the heart to deliver blood forward to the body. In aortic stenosis, if the impediment to eject blood is substantial, the patient may experience dizziness or even fainting because the heart is unable to deliver adequate amounts of blood and oxygen to the brain. Understandably, this occurs most often when a patient is standing, or especially just after a patient rises from a seated or lying position. This is a sign of severe valve disease.

Aortic stenosis can also manifest the increased load on the left ventricle by producing angina, even in the absence of obstructions of the coronary arteries. The excess work required to push the blood past the stenotic aortic valve increases the heart's demand for blood beyond the delivery capacity of even normal coronary arteries. Again, this is a manifestation of substantial obstruction in the heart valve.

All of the conditions affecting the mitral and aortic valves can cause shortness of breath. This is because the extra loads placed on the left ventricle by mitral and/or aortic valve disease cause the pressures inside the left heart to rise. As these pressures rise, the increase is passed back through the pulmonary veins to the lungs. This increased fluid pressure in the lungs leads to the sensation of shortness of breath. Increased activity, and therefore increased demand for blood, may exacerbate this symptom. When the pressure increase in the lungs is sufficient, fluid may actually leak into the tiny air spaces in the lung. This condition, called pulmonary edema, can cause severe shortness of breath and reduce the oxygen levels in the blood.

Fluid retention can be seen with all valve abnormalities but especially in conditions which overload the right heart and which may also cause tricuspid insufficiency. Fluid overload in these cases is most commonly manifested by swelling in the lower legs, feet, and ankles. As noted, several valve conditions can trigger body reflexes to hold on to fluid in an effort to compensate for inadequate forward delivery of blood. When this fluid retention is significant, swelling of the lower parts of the body may appear since gravity pulls this extra fluid down during the day. Often the swelling, called edema, will be worse at the end of the day and will be diminished or absent in the morning. This is because of the action of gravity when the patient is awake and upright, and the re-absorption of the edema fluid at night when the patient's feet are at the same level as his heart.

Clearly, a great variety of cardiac conditions can produce important symptoms. On the basis of these symptoms, and even with careful physical examination, it may not be possible to define accurately the precise abnormalities of the patient's cardiac condition. For this reason, sophisticated diagnostic testing procedures have been developed. These tests will be described in the following chapters. ♥

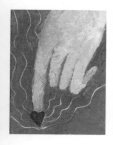

CHAPTER 5

# Echocardiography and Other Non-invasive Tests

*In order to better define abnormalities* of heart structure and function, a number of non-invasive diagnostic tests have been developed. Non-invasive refers to the fact that the test can be performed, and the information obtained, without the need to enter a body space with a needle or to make an incision with a scalpel. The most useful non-invasive diagnostic tests include echocardiography, exercise and other forms of stress testing, and radionuclide cardiac scanning. In this chapter, we will also review ultra fast CT scanning (sometimes called electron beam CT scanning, or "heart scanning") and cardiac magnetic resonance imaging (MRI).

Echocardiography is one of the most useful diagnostic tests in modern cardiology. An echocardiogram is performed using sound waves like SONAR on a submarine. An instrument (transducer) that can both send and receive sound waves is used to obtain the signals that are computer processed to make images of the cardiac structures and the blood flowing through them. These images can be obtained by placing the transducer on the outside of the chest and aiming it at the heart. This is called a transthoracic echocardiogram. A special gel is used to obtain good acoustical contact

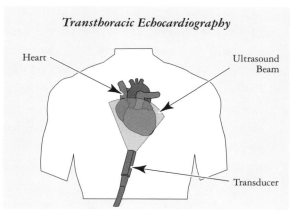

**Transthoracic Echocardiography**

Heart

Ultrasound Beam

Transducer

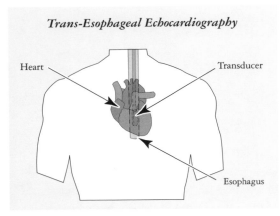

**Trans-Esophageal Echocardiography**

Heart

Transducer

Esophagus

between the transducer and the skin when a transthoracic echo is performed. Alternatively, specialized transducers can be placed in the esophagus (swallowing tube) of a sedated and locally-anesthetized patient, and images obtained from a vantage point behind the heart.

This view is particularly useful for examining the mitral valve since the left atrium, and therefore the mitral valve, sits just in front of the esophagus.

Two kinds of information are available from echocardiograms. The easiest to understand are the images that can be obtained of the heart muscle and chambers and of the valves. These images are in two dimensions. The way to think about this is to imagine that the echo transducer is a knife making a slice through the heart. The angle of the transducer determines the angle at which the sound waves "slice" the heart and therefore the angle of the cross-sectional picture that is obtained. Various parts of the heart from various angles therefore can be observed by moving, and/or angling, the transducer.

Echocardiographic images give information about the thickness of the heart muscle and how well it moves. Deviations from normal are useful in understanding both the cause of a patient's symptoms and the underlying cardiac disease. In addition to information about the muscle itself, the echocardiogram also provides an image of the size and shape of the various chambers of the heart. Certain conditions can cause enlargement of cardiac chambers or show that all, or part of the wall, of the heart is not contracting well. This information, too, can be useful in understanding the nature of a patient's heart disease.

Among the most useful information obtainable from the

echocardiogram is that about the structure and the function of the cardiac valves, particularly the aortic and mitral valves. As noted, the transesophageal echocardiogram gives particularly good information about the mitral valve. The echocardiographic images provide information about the thickness and mobility of the valves, the presence of calcification, the size of a stenotic valve orifice, and whether there is prolapse of one or more of the valve leaflets. This information can be crucial in making a precise diagnosis of a patient's heart condition. It is also extremely important to the surgeon in planning operative correction of valve problems, particularly when a valve repair is planned.

Intra-operative use of transesophageal echocardiography has become an indispensable tool of the cardiac surgeon. As noted, this imaging technique gives detailed information about the cardiac structures, especially the mitral valve. In the operating room, the transesophageal echocardiogram is used to define the abnormal anatomy precisely so that an effective operation can be planned. After the operation is complete, but while the patient is still in the operating room, the echocardiogram can confirm the efficacy of the operation or identify residual abnormalities that must be corrected.

Other intra-operative uses of the echocardiogram include examination of the ascending and other parts of the aorta. This can be done with the transesophageal echo transducer, or with a hand-held transducer placed in a sterile bag and applied directly to cardiac structures. Examination of the aorta is important in identifying atherosclerotic disease of this blood vessel. This is important since most cardiac operations require some manipulation of the aorta and avoidance of disruption of diseased segments of the aorta is important.

Another important examination of the aorta for which echocardiography is useful is in the identification of aortic dissection (see Chapter 12). Aortic dissection is a catastrophic acute disease of the aorta. Because of its outstanding imaging capabilities, transesophageal echocardiography is one of the diagnostic modalities of choice for identifying aortic dissection.

The echocardiogram also provides information about the flow

of blood through the heart. This information helps to make the diagnosis of both stenosis and insufficiency of the aortic and mitral valves. Valve abnormalities create abnormalities of blood flow that can be identified by the specific patterns that are made on echo flow studies.

Stenotic valves cause accelerations in the flow of blood past them since the heart must push blood through a narrower opening in a relatively limited amount of time. Using the Doppler principal (the frequency of sound waves changes related to the velocity with which the source is moving toward or away from the observer) the speed of blood flow past a valve can be measured. Formulas have been developed that can relate these speeds to the pressure drop across the valve. This pressure drop is related to the severity of obstruction of a stenotic valve.

Valve insufficiency also causes abnormalities of blood flow that can be detected echocardiographically. When a valve leaks, the blood flows in the wrong direction at certain times in the cardiac cycle. This abnormal blood flow can be detected — again based on the physics of the Doppler effect. Also, flow around an abnormal valve is turbulent, not the smooth flow that is characteristic of normal structures. This turbulent flow can be visualized by echocardiography. The computer that processes the echo signals can turn information about flow direction and turbulence into specific colors based on whether the blood is moving toward or away from the transducer. Such color Doppler images give important information about the nature and magnitude of valve dysfunctions.

There are varieties of ways to perform stress testing, but all seek the same information. The primary question addressed by a stress test is whether there is heart muscle that is not receiving adequate amounts of blood. A second, related kind of information available from stress tests performed with radioactive dyes is whether there are certain areas of the heart that are scarred or other areas that are alive, but with baseline inadequate blood flow.

The simplest kind of stress test is performed by having a patient exercise on a treadmill while the electrocardiogram is being

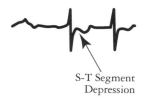

*EKG Changes That May Mean a Positive Stress Test*

S-T Segment Depression

S-T Segment Depression

monitored. The patient proceeds through graded levels of exercise. The test is terminated when the patient reaches a predicted maximum heart rate based on age. The test is only considered valid if the patient reached 80 percent of this predicted peak heart rate. The test may be terminated earlier by patient fatigue, if the patient develops symptoms consistent with angina, or if there are changes on the electrocardiogram suggesting that the patient's heart is not getting enough blood. The location of changes on the electrocardiogram also can pinpoint, relatively accurately, the part of the heart not getting enough blood and therefore suggest which artery may be involved.

All of these endpoints yield potentially important information about the possible presence of coronary artery disease with obstructions severe enough that inadequate blood is available to supply the heart muscle under conditions of increased demand. The limitations of this test stem from the fact that patients may have significant decrements of heart blood flow without either symptoms or typical EKG changes. Furthermore, some EKG changes, even when present, are non-specific and do not make a definitive diagnosis of coronary artery disease. Interestingly, it turns out that the accuracy of exercise stress testing is somewhat dependent on the likelihood that the patient tested actually has heart disease. In other words, in a group of patients with significant risk factors for coronary artery disease the chance that the test will accurately predict who has disease and who does not is measurably higher than if a group of patients with few or no risk factors is tested. This is why this test is not usually recommended as a screening test for the general population.

Combining this test with heart muscle scanning can increase the accuracy of exercise testing. A heart scan is performed by injecting a chemical that emits small amounts of radiation that can be detected by a camera, analogous to a Geiger counter. The chemical most often used is a radioactive isotope called thallium. Thallium shares properties with potassium, an electrically charged particle. Potassium is normally found inside cells in the body; and thallium, when injected, goes where potassium goes — as long as there is a blood supply to deliver the thallium to the cells. When a patient with coronary artery disease exercises, the areas of heart muscle with inadequate blood supply get less thallium delivered. When the camera is subsequently placed over the patient's chest and heart, the image of the heart obtained subsequently has a gap or hole in the area of reduced blood supply.

When patients are unable to exercise, thallium stress imaging can be performed in other ways. The two most common methods used to "stress" the heart involve giving the patient medications that either accelerate and augment heart action (analogous to exercise) or that change the dynamics of blood flow to the heart. A medicine called dobutamine is sometimes given to simulate the effects of exercise on the heart. Dobutamine increases the heart rate and the strength of contraction similar to what happens during exercise. Dobutamine-thallium scanning can detect, therefore, areas of reduced blood perfusion just like exercise-thallium testing can.

Another way to do stress testing is by giving a medicine called persantine. Persantine causes regional increases in heart muscle blood flow. If there are coronary artery obstructions, the blood flow to heart regions beyond these obstructions cannot increase in response to Persantine the way blood flow to unobstructed regions can. The subsequent "holes" on scanning identify the presence of coronary obstructions and the regions involved.

Dobutamine-echocardiography stress testing is another method used to detect the likely presence of coronary artery disease. This test is performed by giving dobutamine while monitoring the echocardiogram. At low doses, dobutamine will increase the heart rate and the strength of contraction of the heart muscle. These changes can be seen on the echocardiogram. As the dose of dobutamine is increased, the heart rate and strength of contraction continue to increase. These increases also increase the heart's demand for blood. When there is coronary artery obstruction, the heart muscle in affected regions is unable to receive adequate blood and oxygen to meet its needs and its strength of contraction will actually increase. This pattern of initial increase followed by subsequent decrease in contraction suggests the presence of coronary artery disease.

One limitation of all of these imaging methods designed to detect coronary artery disease is that they depend on there being a difference in blood perfusion between different areas of the heart. In patients with the most severe forms of coronary artery disease, all three coronary vessels are affected and the blood supply to the entire heart is in potential jeopardy. In these cases, the imaging modalities described above may not detect decrements in blood supply since there is no contrast between one region and the other. This is why the search for accurate screening tests for coronary artery disease continues.

A relatively new screening test is the heart scan, or ultra-fast CT scan. A CT scan is a computer-processed image derived from multiple X-ray images taken from different angles. The heart scan is a CT scanner that acquires the multiple images sufficiently rapidly to create a picture of a moving structure like the heart. The heart scan does not provide a picture of the coronary arteries themselves and cannot determine whether there is significant obstruction in them. The heart scan detects only the presence of calcium in the walls of the coronary arteries. There is a relationship between the amount of calcium in the coronary arteries, the calcium "score," and the probability that a patient has significant coronary artery obstructions. A patient with a score of 0 has a very low risk of CAD. A patient with a high score has a high risk. The ultimate diagnosis of CAD still depends, however, on obtaining a picture of the inside of the vessels themselves. This requires an invasive procedure called cardiac catheterization and coronary angiography.

Before we turn to catheterization, however, it is worth considering multi-slice CT scans and cardiac magnetic resonance imaging (MRI). New CT scanners can take such detailed images that visualization of the coronary arteries is now possible. Using this technology, it is feasible also to create images of obstructions in the coronary arteries without the need for catheterization. This capability is not yet widely available, nor has its accuracy been proven. Nonetheless, it may offer the possibility of making an accurate diagnosis without the risks and discomfort of catheterization.

Similarly, cardiac MRI remains for now largely a research tool and is still under development as a clinical diagnostic test. MRI, however, also has the promise of sufficient resolution to produce actual pictures of blood vessels (angiograms) as small as coronary arteries (1-3 mm). Cardiac MRI can also be synchronized with the heartbeat to give spectacularly detailed pictures of the heart muscle walls, the valves, and blood flowing through the heart. As cardiac MRI is perfected, it may allow a whole new level of diagnostic accuracy and precision. And, it is a non-invasive test. ♥

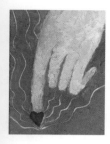

CHAPTER 6

# Cardiac Catheterization

*The first heart catheterization* was done by a physician on himself in the 1930s. This pioneer threaded a catheter through his own arm vein and into his heart. He then walked to the X-ray department and confirmed that he had placed the end of the catheter in his heart by getting a chest X-ray. The more modern techniques used in cardiac catheterization today were developed and perfected relatively recently — in the 1960s — by doctors in several institutions.

Cardiac catheterization is an invasive diagnostic and some-

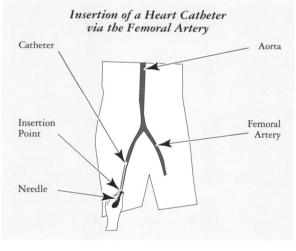

*Insertion of a Heart Catheter via the Femoral Artery*

Catheter

Aorta

Insertion Point

Femoral Artery

Needle

times therapeutic procedure. This is done with an awake-but-sedated patient and local anesthesia. Catheterization involves puncturing an artery and a vein (usually in the groin) with a needle and then intro-ducing various catheters into the blood vessels over a wire passed through the needles. A catheter is a long thin tube that can be used both to measure pressure in the area at its tip and through which special dyes can be injected which allow visualization by X-ray of the inside of structures. Sometimes catheterization is done through blood vessels in the arm near the elbow or even at the wrist.

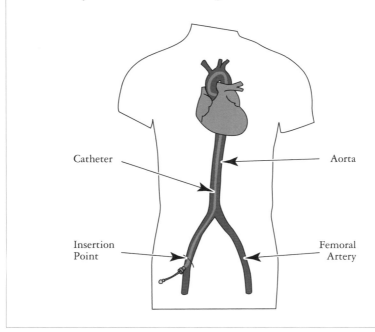

*Path of a Heart Catheter through the Aorta and into the Heart*

Catheter

Aorta

Insertion Point

Femoral Artery

The catheters that are inserted are visible using special X-ray cameras that can show a continuous, moving X-ray picture, and also can make X-ray movies that are recorded. The recordings used to be on 35-mm film but modern catheterization laboratories now use digital storage on CDs, or in digital image archives. Under X-ray guidance, the catheters are passed through the blood vessels of the body to where they can be positioned in various chambers of the heart or at the orifices of the coronary arteries where they come off the aorta. Once in position, the catheters can measure the pressures in various parts of the heart or be used to take pictures of the chambers of the heart, especially the left ventricle, the coronary arteries, and the ascending aorta.

Pressures can be measured in either the right or the left side of the heart. The right-sided pressures are obtained by passing catheters through veins and into the right atrium, the right ventricle, and the pulmonary artery. Abnormal pressures in these areas can be a

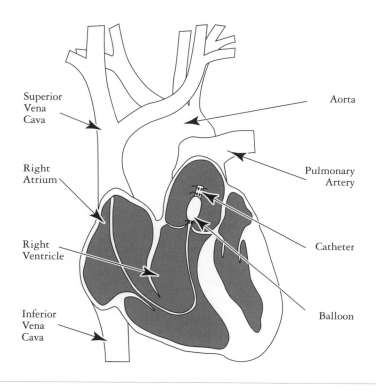

*Pulmonary Artery Catheter*

Superior Vena Cava

Aorta

Right Atrium

Pulmonary Artery

Right Ventricle

Catheter

Inferior Vena Cava

Balloon

sign of significant disease on the left side of the heart. Also, intrinsic lung disease can be manifest by elevated right-sided pressures. In addition, special catheters can be introduced into the right heart to measure the function of the heart. Various techniques are used to assess cardiac output, the volume of blood that the heart circulates, measured in liters per minute. The normal cardiac output at rest in an adult is about 5 L/min.

Catheters on the left side of the heart can be advanced retrograde through the aorta and across the aortic valve and into the left ventricle. The mitral valve cannot be crossed using this method. Left atrial pressures can be measured directly by puncture across the septum separating the right from the left atrium, but this technique is used rarely today. The pressure drop across a diseased, narrowed (stenotic)

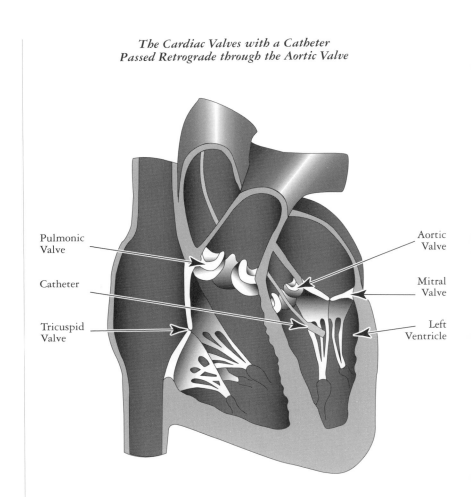

**The Cardiac Valves with a Catheter
Passed Retrograde through the Aortic Valve**

Pulmonic
Valve

Catheter

Tricuspid
Valve

Aortic
Valve

Mitral
Valve

Left
Ventricle

mitral valve can be measured indirectly by simultaneously measuring a pulmonary artery wedge pressure and the left ventricular pressure. The pulmonary artery wedge pressure is obtained by "wedging" a balloon at the tip of the catheter into a branch pulmonary artery. By effectively excluding the main pulmonary pressure from the measurement, the wedge pressure provides an indirect assessment of the left atrial pressure.

More commonly, the left-sided catheter is used to measure left ventricular and aortic pressure. Simultaneous recordings, or a pull back recording in which the catheter is pulled back from the left ventricle to the aorta, can detect and measure accurately the pressure drop across a stenotic aortic valve.

Another important measurement obtained with the ventricular catheter is an assessment of the pressure in the chamber at the end of diastole, the relaxed state of the heart right before it starts to contract. In various disease states, the left ventricular end diastolic pressure is elevated. This measurement gives insight into the extent and severity of heart dysfunction.

Finally, dye can be injected into the left ventricle through this catheter. A cine X-ray recording of the heart during this dye injection gives a picture of how well the heart ejects blood with each beat. By taking measurements from still pictures during ventricular ejection, it is possible to measure the size of the ventricular cavity both at the end of contraction (systole) and the end of filling (diastole). The ratio between the estimated volume (actually it is an area that is calculated from the two-dimensional image) of the heart in systole and diastole is called the ejection fraction.

Stated more simply, the ejection fraction is the percentage of blood in the filled heart that is ejected with each beat. A normal ejection fraction is 60-70 percent. Diseases of the heart muscle (including coronary artery disease) or heart valve problems can cause failure of the heart muscle and reduction of ventricular ejection fraction. Moderate impairment is associated with ejection fractions of 30-40 percent. Severely damaged ventricles may have ejection fractions as low as 10-15 percent.

*Ejection Fraction, a Measure of the Strength of Heart Function*

Diastole (filled) — Left Ventricle

Systole (emptied) — Left Ventricle

The other primary objective of cardiac catheterization is coronary angiography. In this procedure, specialized catheters are engaged in the orifices at the origins of either the left or the right coronary artery. X-ray dye injected into these catheters produces a moving picture of the inside of the vessel allowing a determination of the extent and location of any coronary artery obstructions. Not all obstructions are severe enough to limit blood flow. Most cardiologists and surgeons consider obstructions greater than 60 percent to be severe enough to limit flow. Lesser degrees of obstruction are potentially important, however. First, any degree of obstruction, by definition, means that the patient has coronary artery disease and needs to be monitored and treated as such. Second, as we discussed earlier, sometimes plaques that produce lesser degrees of obstruction are vulnerable to the rupture that can produce a total obstruction and an acute heart attack.

Angioplasty and stenting, catheter-based procedures used to treat coronary artery obstructions essentially utilize the same techniques used to make the pictures of the coronary arteries. Specialized catheters with balloons and/or stents at their tips are used in these therapeutic procedures, which will be described in the next chapter. ♥

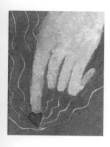

# CHAPTER 7

# Angioplasty and Stents

*Angioplasty is a catheter procedure* to open blocked arteries. The first angioplasties of the coronary arteries were done in the late 1970s. Application of this procedure has grown rapidly along with the development of the technologies to support and extend its utilization.

Coronary angioplasty is done in the catheterization laboratory, like cardiac catheterization, with the patient sedated and under local anesthesia. Access to the blood vessels is through the groin or arm, as in the diagnostic procedures described in Chapter 6. Angioplasty and the other procedures described in this chapter are considered "interventional" procedures since the intent is to intervene to correct a disease process. This is in contra-distinction to "diagnostic" catheterization procedures, which only detect the presence of a disease and do not attempt to treat it.

The angioplasty procedure, as first developed, involved threading a catheter into the orifice of one of the coronary arteries as described previously. Through a special version of such a catheter, a thin "guide" wire is passed into the coronary artery. To do angioplasty, it is crucial that this guide wire be able to be passed beyond the obstruction (this is called "crossing" the lesion or diseased area). If the obstruction cannot be crossed, the procedure cannot be done. Once the guide wire is in place, a catheter with a balloon at its tip is introduced along the wire under X-ray guidance. Using markers on the balloon that are visible by X-rays, the balloon is positioned at the site of obstruction. Once the balloon is positioned, it is inflated under high pressure for a limited period. Multiple inflations, or

# *Balloon Angioplasty*

Plaque     Balloon     Artery

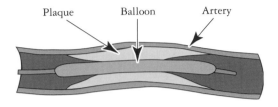

Balloon is positioned in blocked area.

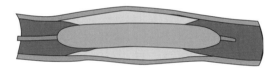

Balloon is inflated, flattening the plaque.

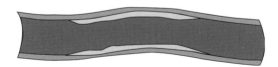

Larger opening is created.

inflations with progressively larger balloons, are performed.

The result of this procedure is to stretch or even tear the vessel in such a way that the obstruction is relieved. Ideal obstructions are relatively symmetrical and limited in length, but with advances in balloon technology and the stents to be described, the spectrum of types of obstructions that can be dilated has increased.

In the early days of angioplasty, this procedure would lead to worsening of the obstruction, including even total obstruction, in as many as 20 percent of patients. This would require emergency bypass surgery to restore blood flow and prevent a possibly fatal heart attack. Again, due to technological advances including stents, this event is exceedingly rare today.

Even if the balloon dilation procedure is successful initially, about one-third of patients suffer from re-narrowing within six months of the procedure. This requires either repeat angioplasty or bypass surgery.

Examination revealed two processes that contribute to re-narrowing after balloon angioplasty. The first is due to "elastic recoil" of the tissues in the blood vessels. All blood vessels contain tissues with elasticity that tends to restore them to a certain shape and configuration. Elastic recoil after angioplasty is a common cause of early restenosis. The second cause of re-narrowing is tissue over-growth. Balloon angioplasty produces an injury to a blood vessel. Healing cells grow in the vessel in response to this injury. In some patients, this growth of tissue is enough to cause a re-obstruction in the artery.

Intra-coronary stents were developed to deal with both abrupt, early closure during the procedure, and with the elastic recoil process. A stent is a small, cylindrical, metal mesh. It is delivered to the site of obstruction in a collapsed state over a catheter with a small balloon inside. The balloon inside the stent has X-ray markers to ensure accurate location of the stent. Once in place, the balloon is inflated, expanding the stent within the coronary artery.

This innovation has all but eliminated abrupt artery closure during the procedure in the catheterization laboratory, and therefore,

## Angioplasty with Stent

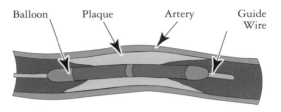

Balloon  Plaque  Artery  Guide Wire

The stent is positioned in the blockage.

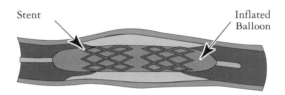

Stent  Inflated Balloon

The balloon is inflated and the stent expands.

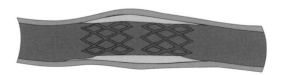

The stent remains in place keeping the artery open.

essentially eliminated emergency bypass surgery following failed angioplasty. This now occurs in less than one percent of cases. Intra-coronary stents have also significantly reduced the rate of re-narrowing within six months of the angioplasty procedure. That is because the stents reduce the tendency of elastic recoil to cause re-development of coronary artery obstructions. The risk of this has now been reduced to about 15-20 percent.

Despite this advance, however, re-narrowing due to overgrowth of healing cells persists as an important limitation of the efficacy of angioplasty and stenting. The newest versions of intra-coronary stents, released in 2003, now have a coating of medicine on their metallic surfaces. These coated stents (as opposed to what are now called "bare metal stents") are sometimes referred to as drug-eluting stents since the medicine in the coating is embedded in a material that releases the medicine slowly (known as eluting) over time.

There are currently two such coated stents being used in patients. Both stents have medicines that inhibit the growth of new cells in the area of the stent. Since the amount of medicine released is small, its effects are local and the drug, therefore, has no known effect on the patient overall.

Although experience with drug-eluting stents is still early, and therefore limited, the efficacy of this innovation seems to be dramatic. In the earliest studies, there was essentially no observation of coronary artery re-narrowing. Subsequent larger studies have shown that there remains a rate of restenosis somewhere in the 5-10 percent range. Whether this advantage will persist long-term, or whether the drug coating merely delays, rather than prevents, re-narrowing, will require more time to demonstrate.

Angioplasty and stenting can be applied to re-open a suddenly obstructed vessel that is causing a heart attack. In this setting, the procedure is usually called "primary angioplasty." Before the development of reliable stents, patients who came to the hospital in the midst of an acute heart attack either received no treatment to the attack or were given "clot busting" drugs to try to dissolve the clot that was obstructing the coronary artery.

With present technology and techniques, however, it is now possible to completely re-open totally obstructed arteries that are causing heart attacks. These primary angioplasties must be accomplished expeditiously, since "time is muscle." In order to prevent irreversible damage to the heart, a completed heart attack, the artery should be opened within two hours or less from the time the patient presents to the hospital. While this requires exquisite co-ordination between the ambulance crew, the emergency department and the catheterization laboratory, it can be accomplished reliably with suitably trained and prepared teams. When primary angioplasty is accomplished, heart muscle is preserved, heart attacks are aborted, and lives are saved.

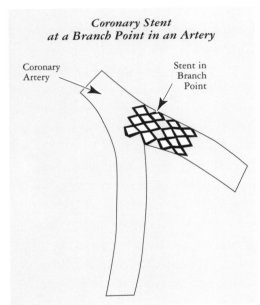

*Coronary Stent at a Branch Point in an Artery*

Coronary Artery

Stent in Branch Point

Since these catheter interventional procedures are so effective and increasingly durable, why doesn't every patient have angioplasty and stenting rather than undergoing bypass surgery? Unfortunately, not every patient is a candidate for angioplasty. Some patients have disease in their vessels that is too diffuse or involves areas that are inaccessible to the guide wire or at branch points. Branch point narrowings can be a problem since placing a stent in one branch may compromise the other. Most cardiologists are reluctant to use stents in the left main coronary artery. This is because the left main is a short vessel and accurate placement of the stent may be difficult. Also, the left main supplies blood to a large part of the heart. Any problem with the procedure might have catastrophic consequences if the blood supply to much of the heart were suddenly obstructed. In some patients, especially in situations where the artery to be treated is totally obstructed, the guide wire cannot be passed beyond the obstruction. As mentioned, failure to cross the narrowing makes the procedure impossible.

These considerations mean that there must remain an option beyond angioplasty for patients whose coronary artery disease cannot be managed successfully with medicines. Heart surgery is that option. Coronary bypass surgery, the operative treatment of coronary artery disease, will be described in Chapter 9. We will precede this with a brief discussion of the heart-lung machine, an important tool used in most cardiac surgery operations. ♥

# The Heart-Lung Machine and its Attachments to the Heart

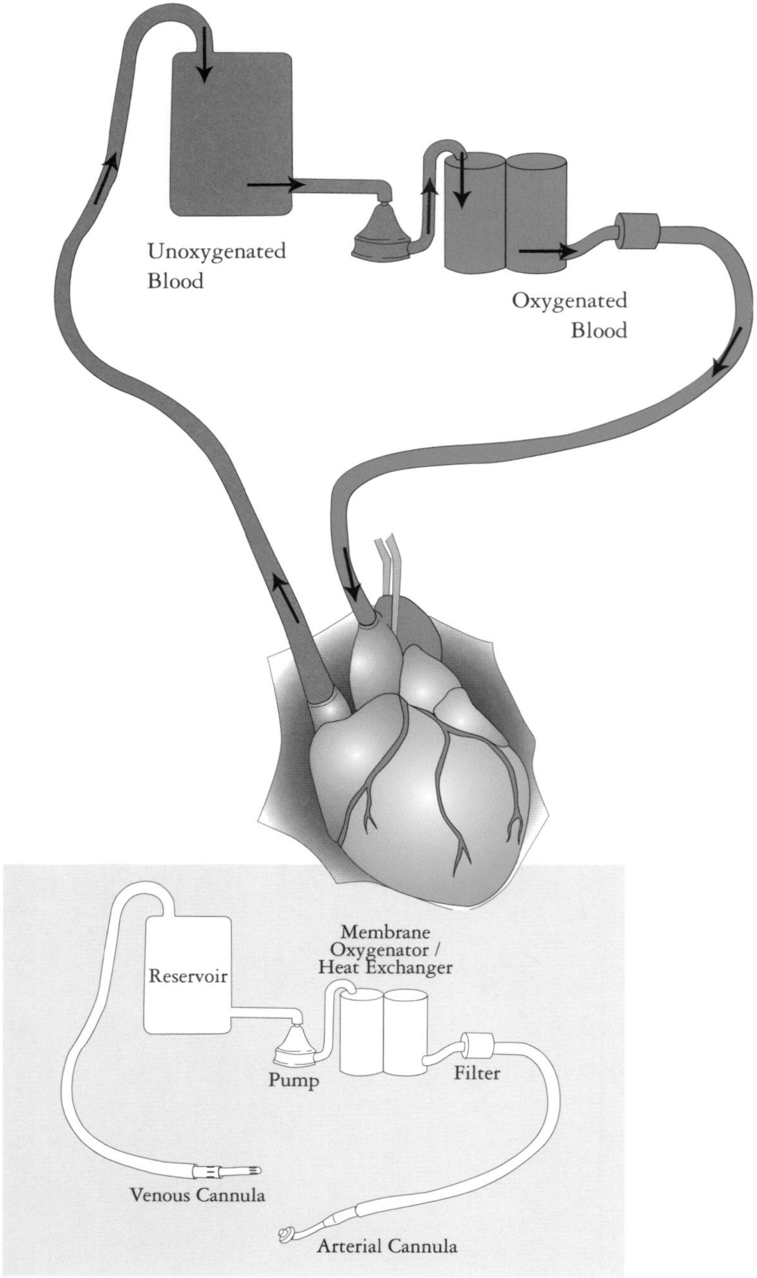

Unoxygenated Blood

Oxygenated Blood

Reservoir

Membrane Oxygenator / Heat Exchanger

Pump

Filter

Venous Cannula

Arterial Cannula

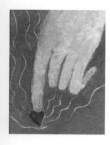

# CHAPTER 8

# The Heart-Lung Machine

*In the 1930s,* a surgeon named John Gibbon, in training at the Massachusetts General Hospital in Boston, sat up all night tending to a dying patient with a pulmonary embolus (a blood clot that travels from a leg vein to the pulmonary artery). The patient died, but all during that night, Dr. Gibbon reasoned that if only he had a machine that would temporarily do the job of the heart and lungs, the patient might have survived. He spent the next twenty years of his life developing a heart-lung machine and used it successfully in 1953 to repair a congenital defect in a young woman's heart.

Other pioneers in cardiac surgery contributed to the development of this device, which temporarily does the jobs of both the heart and the lungs. In the simplest terms, the heart is a pump that pushes blood to the lungs for oxygen and then out to the rest of the body to deliver the oxygen. The lungs put the oxygen in the blood. These are the two basic functions of the heart-lung machine: to put oxygen in the blood and to pump the oxygenated blood throughout the body.

The details of the technology are much more complicated, and there have been tremendous advances in the sophistication and safety of the heart-lung machine in the fifty years since Gibbon's first success. The heart-lung machine is sometimes called a cardiopulmonary (cardio = heart, pulmonary = lung) bypass or simply *a bypass machine*, since it makes it possible for the circulation to almost completely bypass (avoid passing through) the heart and the lungs.

Why is this important? In order to perform operations inside the heart, it is necessary to stop the circulation of blood through the heart and lungs so that the heart can be opened and work performed inside the heart. Also, for coronary bypass surgery, which is done on the surface of the heart without opening it, cardiopulmonary bypass allows the surgeon to operate on small arteries (1-3 mm) on a still heart without blood in the vessels obscuring the view. (We will discuss this, and off-pump bypass surgery, in the next chapter.) The heart-lung machine keeps the body alive by maintaining the oxygenation and the circulation of blood while the heart and lungs are quiescent.

Patients are temporarily attached to a heart-lung machine by the insertion of specialized cannulas (tubes) into the heart. A large cannula is placed, either in the right atrium, or in both the superior and inferior venae cavae, in order to drain unoxygenated blood from the patient and into the heart-lung machine. The blood then passes through an oxygenator, essentially an artificial lung, in which oxygen is added and carbon dioxide removed. There has been a lot of progress in the efficiency and safety of oxygenators over the years. Early oxygenators bubbled oxygen through the blood. This process is damaging to blood cells and creates the need to remove the bubbles and foam that inevitably accumulate in the blood before the blood is pumped back into the patients. Modern oxygenators consist of fine capillaries (very small tubes) that allow oxygen to diffuse through their walls so that there is no damaging direct contact between blood and oxygen.

After being oxygenated, the blood usually passes through a filter to remove particulate matter and gas before it is pumped back to the patient. The blood usually re-enters the patient's circulation by a cannula placed at the top of the ascending aorta, although sometimes this cannula is placed in another artery such as the femoral artery in the groin or the axillary artery by the shoulder. Medications can be given to the patient through the bypass circuit to maintain anesthesia, or to ensure that the patient's blood pressure is in the proper range. Most heart-lung machine pumps do not provide a pulsatile flow of blood (with a systolic and a diastolic pressure as the normal circulation) so it is the mean pressure that the perfusionist, a specially trained clinician who runs the heart-lung machine, tries to maintain in the normal range.

Another important function of the heart-lung machine is to deliver what is called cardioplegia solution to the patient's heart. Cardioplegia literally means "heart paralysis" and the purpose of this solution is to stop the heart in a relaxed state and to cool it in order to prevent damage when the heart is deprived of blood. In order to operate on the heart, it is necessary to prevent blood from passing through it. This not only means the blood that passes through the heart's pumping chambers, but also the blood in the coronary arteries that nourish the heart. In order not to damage the heart during surgery, which can range from twenty minutes in simple operations, to as much as two to three hours in the most complex procedures, cardioplegia solution is administered to the heart via the coronary arteries.

Cardioplegia is a blood-based solution that contains oxygen, which is delivered in the blood that also provides a buffer against the build-up of acid and other waste products. Additional potassium is added to the solution. High doses of potassium stop the heart in a relaxed state. A relaxed heart requires less oxygen to stay alive and therefore is better able to tolerate the temporary deprivation of blood. The final important active ingredient in most cardioplegia solutions is cold. The heart is cooled to as low as 12 degrees Centigrade. A cold heart also needs less oxygen and energy to stay alive, and therefore is less subject to damage during the period of time that the heart is stopped and deprived of blood. Most surgeons give intermittent doses of cardioplegia solution to protect the heart during an operation and provide an unobstructed view of the intra-cardiac structures. Some advocate continuous infusion of cardioplegia, which nevertheless must be stopped from time to time so that the cardioplegia blood does not obscure the operative field.

Despite the tremendous contribution of the heart-lung machine and cardiopulmonary bypass, there are complications and side effects associated with its use. The insertion of cannulas and manipulation of the aorta sometimes dislodge atherosclerotic debris, or blood clots, that can float downstream in the circulation and cause damage to the brain (a stroke, for instance ), kidneys, or other organs. Since air enters the heart when it is open, it must be removed when the normal circulation is re-started. Air is poorly soluble in blood and therefore makes bubbles. Unless these bubbles are removed, they can float downstream like blood clots and cause damage to vital organs.

The heart-lung machine also presents a relatively large surface of non-biologic material in contact with blood. This blood-surface contact activates a response of systemic inflammation. This means that blood cells, proteins, and other substances in blood are activated. The activated substances can cause temporary changes in blood vessel and organ function. The changes cause fluid retention in patients after heart surgery and are responsible for adding to a patient's soreness and fatigue after heart surgery.

Finally, to prevent blood clotting during contact with the artificial surfaces of the heart-lung machine, anti-coagulants, blood thinners, are given to patients having heart operations. The anticoagulants are reversed after the surgery but often some residual thinning of the blood remains. Also, the heart-lung machine causes changes in platelets, the small blood cells that promote blood clotting. The clear fluid used to prime the heart-lung machine dilutes all blood cells and substances, including the clotting proteins. These factors mean that all patients are somewhat anemic (having a low red blood count) after heart surgery. This can increase symptoms of post-operative fatigue. There is also a risk of bleeding in the first few hours after a heart operation. This is monitored carefully and occasionally requires a return to the operating room to drain any blood that may accumulate around the heart, and to repair a bleeding point if there is one. This does not require redoing the entire operation, and patients usually make an uneventful recovery.

The heart-lung machine has made modern heart surgery possible. While this device, like any other medical procedure or therapy, has costs, side effects, and complications, its contribution to the care of patients with heart disease, in most cases, far outweighs any disadvantages. ♥

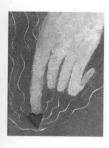

# CHAPTER 9

# Coronary Artery Bypass Surgery

*Coronary artery disease (CAD),* or obstruction to the vessels that supply blood to the heart, is the most common heart condition. By depriving the heart of blood, coronary artery disease can cause chest pain (angina) and heart attacks that can permanently damage the heart muscle. In coronary bypass surgery, the surgeon takes blood vessels from elsewhere in the body and attaches them to the coronary arteries upstream and downstream from the blocked vessel.

*Coronary Bypass Surgery*

Vein Graft

Aorta

Blockage

Internal Mammary Artery Graft

Right Coronary Artery

Left Anterior Descending Coronary Artery

This procedure provides an alternate route or a "bypass" for the blood to get to the heart. Interestingly, various parts of the body can tolerate removal of blood vessels used for the bypasses, since, in most areas, alternative blood vessels exist and take over the job of carrying the blood.

The indications for bypass surgery have been well defined by several studies in patients over the last thirty years. Bypass surgery is extremely effective in relieving the symptoms of CAD. In patients whose symptoms are persistent despite medications, or in those who cannot tolerate medications, or in patients whose lifestyle makes taking medications undesirable, symptoms alone may be an indication for bypass surgery.

The other primary indication for bypass surgery is prevention of heart attack and prolongation of life. Studies have identified several classes of patients in whom bypass surgery both prevents heart attacks and extends life. Patients with significant left main disease are best managed with bypass surgery for this reason. Similarly, it has been shown that patients with three vessel coronary artery disease and impaired left ventricular function do better with bypass surgery. Patients with two coronary arteries obstructed, one of which is the upstream portion of the left anterior descending artery (LAD), have improved survival with bypass surgery. Finally, patients with angina or other evidence of inadequate heart muscle blood flow at rest, especially immediately after a heart attack, are improved with bypass surgery.

Many of the same indications apply to angioplasty and stents (described in Chapter 7), although not all patients with indications for bypass surgery are also candidates for stents (left main, diffuse three-vessel disease, etc.). Many studies have attempted to compare the results of angioplasty and coronary artery bypass grafts (CABG). These consistently show that symptoms recur earlier and more frequently after angioplasty than after bypass surgery. However, patient survival appears not to be different in the long run, with the probable exception of patients with diabetes who appear to do better with surgery.

For bypass surgery, the patient is under general anesthesia. The heart is exposed in nearly all heart operations by an incision down the middle of the chest. The breastbone (sternum) is divided lengthwise in the middle. This incision is called a "median sternotomy."

In the usual procedure, the patient has his heart temporarily attached to the heart-lung machine. The surgeon stops the heart so that the bypass grafts can be sewn accurately to the coronary arteries that can be as small as 1 mm. As noted in Chapter 8, the heart-lung machine can cause complications, especially in patients with other diseases of the brain, lungs, or kidneys. Using new devices that stabilize the heart without stopping it, surgeons can now do bypass operations without the heart-lung machine. In such "beating heart" or "off-pump" surgery, the operation can be done with fewer potential complications. Although not all patients are suitable for this surgery, in the right patients, it can be life saving.

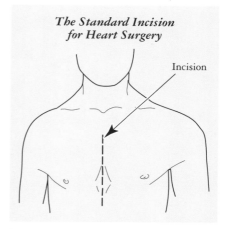

*The Standard Incision for Heart Surgery*

Incision

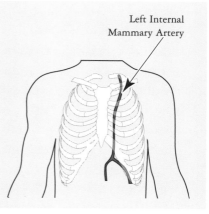

Left Internal Mammary Artery

In almost every bypass operation, the left internal mammary artery is used to graft the left anterior descending artery on the front surface of the heart. The left internal mammary artery is located on the inside of the chest wall just to the left of the sternum. It has been shown that use of this bypass conduit improves the results, measured in patient survival, in both the short-term and the long-term. Mammary artery grafts to the LAD are also the most durable of all the bypass grafts. In a large series of patients, it has been shown that the chance that this graft will still be working in ten years is 90-95 percent.

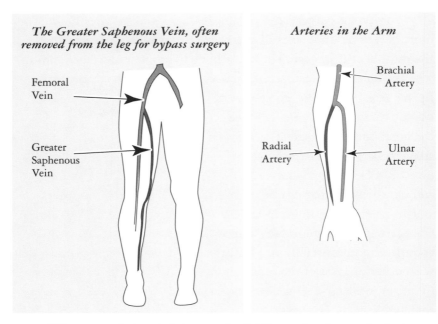

**The Greater Saphenous Vein, often removed from the leg for bypass surgery**

Femoral Vein

Greater Saphenous Vein

**Arteries in the Arm**

Brachial Artery

Radial Artery

Ulnar Artery

When vessels in addition to the LAD need to be grafted, there are several choices of conduits to be used. One of the original bypass conduits—and still the most frequently used—is the greater saphenous vein. This is a superficial leg vein running from the groin down the inner thigh and calf all the way to the ankle. The entire length of this vein can be removed since the body has multiple alternative routes for the blood to be returned from the leg. Each bypass graft requires about eight inches of vein, so multiple grafts can be performed with the saphenous vein, especially if they are linked together in what is called "sequential" grafting.

The saphenous vein is a vein, obviously, and not an artery. The probability that vein grafts will still be open in 10 years has been observed to be about 60 percent. One conclusion is that when veins are used to bypass arteries they are not as durable (compared to mammary artery durability). However, it has been demonstrated that both artery and vein grafts placed on the LAD last longer than grafts placed elsewhere. Many factors appear to be involved. One result of this observation, however, has been increased interest in using all arteries to bypass coronary arteries.

One alternative bypass conduit is the right internal mammary artery. There is some evidence that the use of both the left and the right mammary arteries gives superior long-term survival and freedom from symptoms, consistent with the all-artery hypothesis. However, in diabetic patients use of both mammary arteries may cause an increase in infection and other healing problems in the sternum. The radial artery, located on the thumb side of the inner forearm is used more frequently today. The radial artery affords the possible advantage of using all arteries for this operation without any added risk to the healing of the sternum. However, there is some concern that the radial artery is prone to spasm and possibly early closure in some patients. For these reasons it is still used selectively and patients often take medicines to prevent arterial spasm for several months after surgery.

In low risk patients, bypass surgery has a mortality risk of less than one percent. Heart function is an important risk factor for all heart operations. In patients with poor heart function, the risk may be considerably higher. But, as we will discuss in Chapter 14, bypass surgery can sometimes improve heart function. By definition, patients with CAD have atherosclerosis that can also affect blood vessels in and near the brain. In addition, most bypass operations require some manipulation of the aorta, even if done off-pump. Therefore, stroke is a risk during or after bypass surgery. Fortunately, this risk is usually low, although elderly patients may have risk of stroke as high as 8 percent.

Bleeding, which usually occurs in the first few hours after surgery, and infection, are complications that can happen after any surgical operation. The risk of the former is 1-2 percent—and of the latter less than one percent. With any major operation and general anesthetic, there can be complications of pneumonia or other lung disease, kidney failure, liver injury, or involvement of any organ system in the body. The risk of these complications is quite low unless the patient already has significant underlying disease. In these circumstances, the off-pump approach may have advantages, but the scientific data to prove this do not yet exist.

An important component of any operation on the heart, and for that matter of any hospitalization for heart disease, is a post-operative and post-discharge plan for cardiac rehabilitation. Along with prevention, diagnosis, and treatment, rehabilitation comprises a key component of proper management of cardiovascular disease. Many hospitals and heart centers have formal programs in cardiac rehabilitation and most patients can benefit from at least several weeks of graded, supervised activity. The amount of formal rehabilitation required depends on the patient's state of debility and the need for a formalized structure to maintain consistency of participation.

In the long term, patients have excellent relief of symptoms, and in certain patients, the benefits of prolongation of life. Expansion of the application and improvement in the results of angioplasty and stenting appear to be reducing the number of patients referred for bypass surgery. This remains, however, one of the most frequently performed operations that can be life saving in certain individuals. It is an operation that has helped millions of individuals suffering from heart disease and continues to play an important role in managing this health problem. ♥

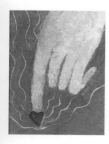

# CHAPTER 10

# Valve Repair

*The best heart valve* is a natural heart valve that functions normally. That is why, especially in the last twenty years, heart surgeons have developed techniques to preserve and repair valves. Most aortic valve pathology is not amenable to repair; but some cases of aortic insufficiency may be correctable. More often, an attempt is made to preserve the aortic valve when it is intrinsically normal but surrounded by aortic pathology (aneurysm, dissection; see Chapter 12) that requires surgery. Mitral stenosis can be repaired, but most cases are too far advanced and valve replacement is necessary. Repair of mitral valve insufficiency is the treatment of choice for this condition and the most commonly performed valve reconstruction.

Aortic insufficiency due to enlargement of one of the leaflets may be amenable to repair by shortening the length of the free margin of the leaflet. This is sometimes a congenital condition, and often the patients who have this operation are quite young. Even if there is involvement of all three aortic valve leaflets, some surgeons will repair the valve by shortening the leaflets at their junction points near the aorta (commissures).

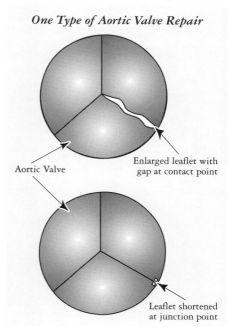

*One Type of Aortic Valve Repair*

Aortic Valve

Enlarged leaflet with gap at contact point

Leaflet shortened at junction point

Such commissural plication may restore competence to the aortic valve in some patients. Attempts to repair calcified, stenotic aortic valves have not met with durable success, and this operation is not done.

The aortic valve may be normal but may be surrounded by diseased aortic tissue that has caused aneurysm or dissection. Dissection, which can disrupt the support of the aortic valve leaflets may be associated with potentially reversible aortic insufficiency. In the past, the operation for disease of the aorta that extended all the way to the aortic valve would have replaced the entire aortic root including the valve. This is no longer the standard operation, although it remains a useful procedure in certain patients.

More often today, surgeons attempt to replace the aorta and preserve the aortic valve. In aortic dissection, often the section of aorta above the valve is replaced and the valve leaflets "re-suspended." This re-suspension restores the normal geometry of the valve, which had been distorted by the disruption of the aorta by the dissection process. Re-suspension can restore normal aortic valve function completely.

*Re-suspension of the Aortic Valve in Aortic Dissection*

Abnormal "unhinged" valve.

Resuspended at each commissure.

Even when the aorta is diseased down to the aortic annulus and requires complete replacement, the aortic valve may be preserved. This requires re-implantation of the valve into the aortic graft. A number of techniques have evolved to perform this re-implantation. One involves sewing the aortic graft to the aortic annulus and then re-attaching the valve commissures and intervening tissues to the wall of the new graft. In the other technique, a scalloped graft is sutured to the aortic remnant just above the valve leaflet tissue. Neither procedure is ideal for all patients.

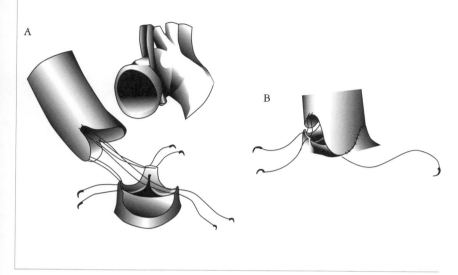

*Re-implantation of the Aortic Valve
During Replacement of the Ascending Aorta*

A

B

One of the issues surrounding this type of valve preservation is the effect that the cylindrical and relatively inelastic graft material may have on aortic valve function. The native aorta has bulges behind each valve leaflet. These "Sinuses of Valsalva" have been shown to play an important role in valve closure by causing a vortex of blood that exerts closing force on the valve leaflets. The long-term effect of loss of these sinuses is not known but may have deleterious consequences for valve function and durability. This has led to the preliminary development of new aortic grafts that have artificial sinuses. These grafts have enlargements at one end that incorporate redundant ridges of Dacron, designed to mimic the elasticity of native sinuses and create the physiologic vortices of blood needed for normal valve closure.

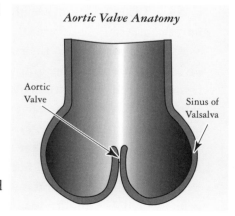

*Aortic Valve Anatomy*

Aortic
Valve

Sinus of
Valsalva

The mitral valve that is stenotic because of rheumatic heart disease may be amenable to repair when the disease is not too severe. It is more likely that the valve can be repaired if there is a lack of significant calcification and scarring and shortening of the chordae tendineae. When the mitral stenosis is due primarily to fusion of the two mitral valve leaflets at their commissures, the valve may be repaired by opening these fused areas. This operation is called a mitral valve commissurotomy. Today mitral commissurotomy can also be accomplished through a catheter technique called balloon mitral valvuloplasty.

*View of Mitral Valve with Stenosis (Narrowing)*

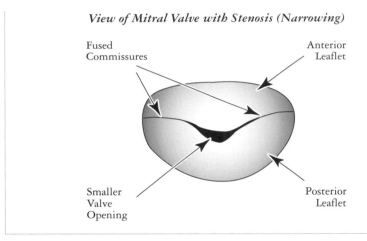

Fused
Commissures

Anterior
Leaflet

Smaller
Valve
Opening

Posterior
Leaflet

This procedure, which is done in the catheterization laboratory under sedation and local anesthesia, requires insertion of catheters into the heart just as described in Chapter 6. Under X-ray guidance, a catheter is passed from the right atrium, across the septum that divides right from left atrium, and across the mitral valve. A special balloon is then positioned across the valve and inflated. This inflation causes tearing of the valve leaflets, usually at the areas of fusion of the commissures. Just as in surgical commissurotomy, this procedure is not done if the patient has a significant amount of mitral insufficiency since this will not get better and may get worse after either type of commissurotomy. In fact, mitral insufficiency is the primary cardiac complication of both these procedures.

Repair of mitral insufficiency not due to rheumatic heart disease is the most commonly performed valve reconstructive operation. It is not usually done for rheumatic mitral insufficiency, since this abnormality is often associated with significant distortion of the mitral apparatus. Most often, mitral valve repair is done for degenerative mitral valve insufficiency. There is a spectrum of these conditions, but all lead to failure of the mitral leaflets to meet and properly maintain competence when the left ventricle contracts.

The normal function of the mitral valve requires the normal function of all its components: annulus, leaflets, and sub-valvar apparatus (chordae and papillary muscles). Any or all may be diseased; and all involved structures must be repaired in order to restore durable valve function. Valve leaflets may lose normal support and all or part of the leaflet may prolapse into the left atrium.

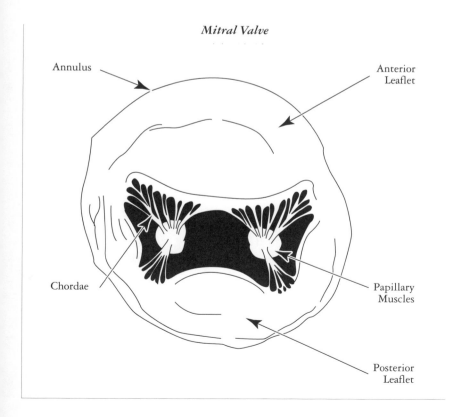

### Mitral Valve

Annulus

Anterior Leaflet

Chordae

Papillary Muscles

Posterior Leaflet

*Types of Leaflet Motion*

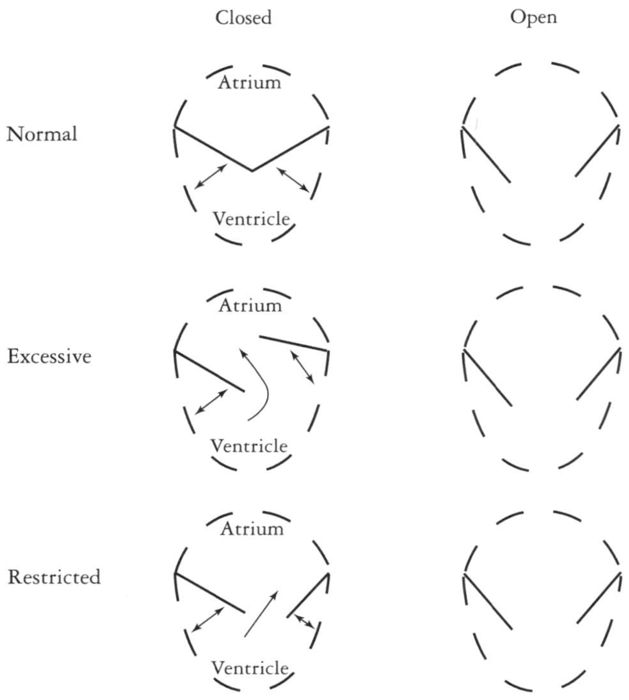

Closed        Open

Normal

Atrium

Ventricle

Excessive

Atrium

Ventricle

Restricted

Atrium

Ventricle

Chordae may be elongated or rupture. These abnormalities lead to abnormal, excessive leaflet motion. The annulus may enlarge, moving the leaflets away from each other. In these cases, leaflet motion is normal but because of the leaflet displacement, the valve leaks. The heart muscle around a papillary muscle may change shape because of a heart attack. This can lead to distortion of the subvalvar apparatus, which restricts the movement of one of the mitral leaflets. This, too, may cause mitral insufficiency. One of the compensatory mechanisms that the body employs is to increase fluid retention when the mitral valve leaks. This leads to increased blood in the heart (since some blood goes backward when there is mitral insufficiency, having more blood in the heart ensures that a more nearly normal amount of blood goes forward). As the heart adapts to this

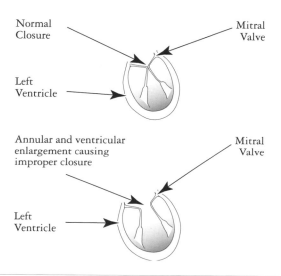

**Changes in Heart Size and Shape
Affect the Function of the Mitral Valve**

Normal
Closure

Mitral
Valve

Left
Ventricle

Annular and ventricular
enlargement causing
improper closure

Mitral
Valve

Left
Ventricle

increased volume load, it enlarges. Enlargement of the heart causes
mitral annular enlargement. This obviously can increase mitral
insufficiency and perpetuate a degenerative cycle.

Effective mitral valve repair requires addressing abnormalities
of the annulus, the leaflets, and the sub-valvar apparatus. Essentially
all mitral valve repairs include
placement of a prosthetic ring
around the mitral annulus. These
rings come in several varieties.
No one design has been proven
superior. The purpose of the
prosthetic ring is to stabilize the
repair. In cases of isolated annular
enlargement, placement of the ring

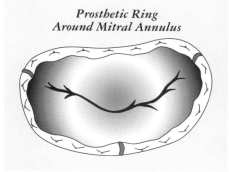

**Prosthetic Ring
Around Mitral Annulus**

is the entire operation. This is because the other functions of the
ring are to restore both normal annular size and the normal shape
of the mitral orifice. Mitral insufficiency can lead to annular
enlargement, which is corrected by the ring.

### Mitral Valve Annuloplasty Ring

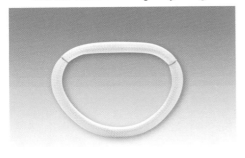

### Mitral Valve Annuloplasty Band

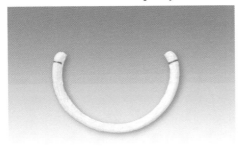

*Images courtesy of Edwards Lifesciences*

An enlarged mitral annulus also has a greater vertical diameter than normal. The ring restores the more asymmetric shape of the mitral annulus by shortening the enlarged area and, with some rings, actively remodeling the shape of the valve orifice.

Prolapsing segments of leaflets may be corrected by actually removing the abnormal portion and simply suturing the valve back together, eliminating the defect. This is most applicable to prolapsing segments of the posterior leaflet. Often anterior or posterior leaflet prolapse is due to chordal elongation or rupture. Techniques available to fix these problems include chordal shortening or chordal transfer from one part of the valve to another. Some surgeons construct artificial chordae from specialized sutures. Other less common techniques include leaflet augmentation (when there is deficient leaflet material as from degeneration or infection) and papillary muscle shortening.

Trans-esophageal echocardiography plays a significant role in the intra-operative care of patients having mitral valve and other valve repairs. The echocardiogram helps define the valve anatomy precisely so that the proper operation can be planned. As important, the echocardiogram is used to assess the valve after repair. No patient should leave the operating room with more than minimal

### Mitral Valve with Abnormality

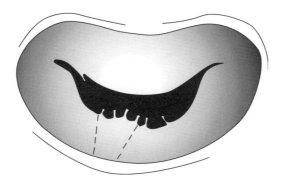

### Abnormal Section Removed

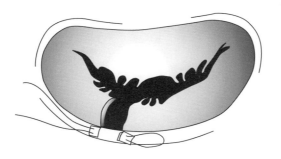

### Valve Sutured Back Together

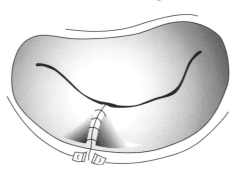

## Transesophageal Echocardiograms

Before mitral valve repair showing large
amount of mitral regurgitation.

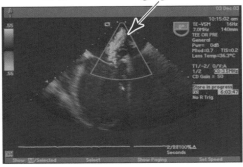

Complete elimination of
regurgitation after valve repair.

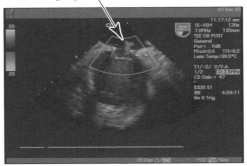

*Images courtesy of Edwards Lifesciences*

residual insufficiency. The long-term efficacy of the repair operation
is dependent on establishing mitral valve competence in the
operating room.

If this is achieved satisfactorily, the durability of mitral valve
repair is excellent. Low rates for re-operation for recurrent valve
insufficiency have been documented out to twenty years. A properly
repaired valve has few complications associated with it, especially
compared to the potential problems with valve prostheses used for
replacement (see Chapter 11). Clearly, the best valve is your own
valve restored to normal function. ♥

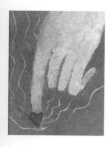

# Valve Replacement

*Valve repair is the preferred procedure* if it is technically feasible, but many patients have valve deformities so advanced that replacement is necessary. There is no ideal replacement device. Each has its own advantages and disadvantages. The various replacement prostheses can be grouped in two major categories: mechanical prostheses made exclusively of non-biologic materials, and tissue valves, which are made of biologic tissues (often animal or human valves), sometimes together with some man-made materials.

Most modern mechanical valves are made of a very hard, metallic appearing substance called pyrolytic carbon. The substance must be durable so that it will not break down despite having to open and close at least 70 times per minute with each heart beat. It must be smooth in order to reduce the risk that it will damage blood cells, or provide a ready surface on which blood clots can form. Modern mechanical valves have either two semi-circular discs, which open and close independently, or a single, circular disk which tilts open and closed. These disks are housed in a ring with a hinge mechanism, which must also be designed for durability and to reduce the risk of clot formation in small nooks and crannies. The ring is covered with synthetic cloth into which the stitches are passed to secure the prosthesis in the valve annulus.

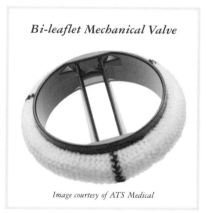

**Bi-leaflet Mechanical Valve**

*Image courtesy of ATS Medical*

All mechanical prostheses have the advantage that they have outstanding durability. Except for the extremely rare event of mechanical disruption and failure, these valves essentially last indefinitely when implanted in humans. They can become infected (any non-biologic device inside the body is subject to this complication) and sometimes the motion of these valves can be obstructed by ingrowth of surrounding tissues. These are the two most common reasons these valves must be replaced. Clotting is the third reason.

The potential for blood clots to form on these valves is their primary disadvantage. Because these prostheses are completely inert biologically, and because they inevitably have small areas of relatively static blood flow, there can be a propensity for blood clots to form on them. Therefore, all patients must take anti-coagulants (blood thinners) indefinitely if they have a mechanical valve implanted. The most commonly used anticoagulant is coumadin, a pill that is taken daily. In order to ensure that the blood is thinned adequately but not excessively, a simple blood test must be done periodically. The name of the test is PT/INR. "PT" stands for "pro-thrombin time," a measure of the clotting activity of the blood. In order to standardize this measurement internationally, the International Normalized Ratio (INR) was developed. The normal PT is 12 seconds and the usual therapeutic range is 18-24 seconds. The normal INR is 1.0 — and after valve replacement, an INR of 2.5-3.5 is usually sought.

The PT/INR must be performed frequently (as often as daily) when coumadin therapy is first started, especially immediately after heart surgery when the patient's diet and activity level have not returned to normal. Once the patient has recovered and is on a stable diet, the frequency at which the PT/INR must be checked may be only monthly. It is possible to lead a relatively normal life on coumadin, although obviously certain activities like contact sports and skydiving are risky because coumadin increases the risk and magnitude of bleeding. Coumadin can be stopped temporarily if the patient needs other surgery, or if there is a bleeding problem. This can be a problem in older patients who may have other conditions that increase the risk of bleeding or which require surgical interventions. The risk of valve clotting or of a blood clot migrating downstream from the valve is about one event for every one hundred patient years. This is often written as 1%/patient-year. In other words, a single patient is at risk for an event every one hundred years. Alternatively, one of every one hundred patients with these valves will have an event each year. This is despite coumadin anticoagulation. There is a similar magnitude risk of unwanted bleeding with coumadin.

The primary advantage of tissue valves is that they do not require lifetime coumadin treatment. Some surgeons prefer that their patients take coumadin for six weeks to three months after tissue valve replacement. After this the blood thinner can be stopped. The main disadvantage of tissue valves is that they can wear out with time. There are two primary failure modes and both are related to the fact that in almost all such prostheses, the tissues have been "fixed" with a chemical and are not alive. Therefore, they have no biological repair mechanisms.

Tissue valves can fail and become incompetent if there is a tear in one or more of the leaflets. This problem is most frequent in the segment of the leaflet near a hinge point. More modern designs have reduced the risk of this sort of failure. Valves may also scar and calcify producing prosthetic valve stenosis sometimes also associated with insufficiency. Again, modern treatment with anti-calcification agents has reduced the risk of this problem.

The propensity for tissue failure is related to age, and also valve position. Tissue valves degenerate more rapidly in younger patients, and this is possibly related to differences in calcium metabolism and immune system activity compared to older patients. Furthermore, older patients, or those with other significant underlying diseases, are likely to have a life expectancy shorter than the projected durability of a tissue valve. For these reasons tissue valves are chosen often in patients over seventy years of age. More recently, surgeons have advocated consideration of tissue valves even in younger patients whose life expectancy may be limited by severe coronary and systemic atherosclerosis, diabetes, or other chronic conditions.

Degeneration of tissue valves is also more frequent in the mitral position than in the aortic position. Essentially all tissue valves are either derived from aortic valves or have a three-leaflet design like the aortic valve. The aortic valve was designed to be closed during the relatively lower pressure of ventricular diastole (relaxation). In the mitral position, the valve must be closed during ventricular systole (contraction) which generates a higher pressure. This additional pressure load, plus the fact that nature's design of the mitral valve is as a two leaflet, rather than a three-leaflet valve, have been hypothesized as the reasons that tissue valves degenerate more rapidly in the mitral position.

In older patients, tissue aortic valves have a 95 percent chance of freedom from structural degeneration at ten years. This probability is lower — about 80 percent — in younger patients. In the mitral position, the probability that the valve will be free of tissue failure at ten years is closer to 60 percent. There is a low risk of blood clots, even without blood thinners with tissue valves.

*Pericardial Valve*

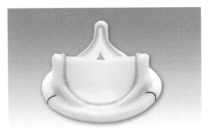

*Stentless Porcine Valve*

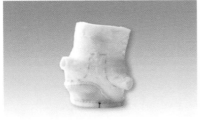

*Images courtesy of Edwards Lifesciences*

Most tissue valves are derived from animal tissues. With the exception of human valves, the tissues in all tissue valves have been "fixed" (tanned) with an organic chemical called glutaraldehyde. This stabilizes the molecular structure of the leaflet tissue.

The first tissue prostheses were constructed from porcine (pig) aortic valves. The earliest designs mounted the porcine valve in a stent, a structure that supported the leaflets. Part of the stent included the sewing ring into which the stitches that secure the valve to the annulus were passed.

The porcine aortic valve is used for both aortic and mitral valve replacements, though less often in the mitral position for the reasons already reviewed.

Newer tissue valves, again used most often for aortic valve replacement, are made from the pericardium (heart sac) of a cow (bovine). Such bovine pericardial valves are completely fabricated. Three leaflets are constructed from pericardium and mounted in a stent. The advantage of this design is better blood flow characteristics compared to the stented porcine valves already described.

The stentless porcine valve is similar to earlier replacement devices which were made from a pig. The porcine valve is made of tanned pig aortic valve tissues. The new stentless valve lacks the man-made struts that support the older versions. These struts take up space and change the action of the valve. The new valves retain the natural porcine aortic wall supports and therefore take up less space. In theory, this means that they may function better, especially in smaller sizes. Furthermore, the lack of struts leads to more normal valve motion that may improve the durability of the new valve. These theoretical advantages need to be proven.

Human heart valves (called "homografts") from patients who have died of other causes, are sometimes used. For obvious reasons, their availability is somewhat limited. These valves are not fixed, but are frozen in a manner designed to try to preserve the viability of the cells in the valves. The evidence that this actually occurs is not convincing. These valves have no non-biologic material and are ideal in situations in which valve replacement is required because of native valve infection. It is hard to prevent or eradicate infection in artificial materials and therefore an all-tissue valve may be advantageous in situations in which there is already infection.

These valves are used most often for aortic valve replacement, although mitral homografts have been implanted. The mitral operation is difficult and the durability of mitral homografts has been poor. The long-term durability of the aortic homograft has been similar to that of porcine and pericardial valves. There is some evidence that the theoretically living frozen homograft has better durability, but these results have not been observed in most centers.

There has been recent interest in an operation called the Ross Procedure, or aortic autograft. In this operation, the patient's own pulmonic valve is removed and used to replace the entire aortic root. A homograft is used to replace the removed pulmonic valve. There is no doubt that the pulmonic autograft is living tissue. For this reason, this operation is indicated in children in whom growth of the aortic valve is important. This rationale is not compelling in full-grown adults. Nevertheless, some surgeons do offer this operation to younger adult patients.

The disadvantages of the Ross Procedure lie in the fact that it is a two-valve operation, with additional associated risks and complications, done for single valve disease. Also, some of the aortic

*Ross Procedure with Aortic Root Replacement*

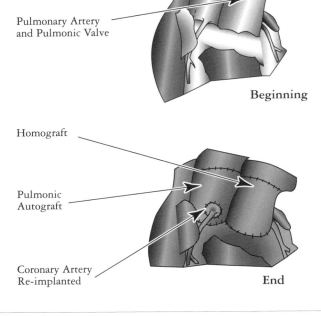

Aorta

Pulmonary Artery
and Pulmonic Valve

**Beginning**

Homograft

Pulmonic
Autograft

Coronary Artery
Re-implanted

**End**

autografts have developed insufficiency over time, severe enough, in some cases, to require re-operation. This seems to be a particular problem when there is a discrepancy in size between the native aortic and pulmonic annuli. Re-operations on the pulmonic homografts also have been required.

Just as after coronary bypass surgery, a program of cardiac rehabilitation is important after any valve operation, repair or replacement. Many patients with valvular heart disease have suffered from chronic disability related to their valve dysfunction and an organized program of increasing activity accelerates their recovery after valve surgery. They come to heart surgery relatively deconditioned, and often more so than the average patient having coronary artery bypass surgery. At least several weeks of formal cardiac rehabilitation is extremely important in helping such patients resume active and productive lives as rapidly as possible following major cardiac surgery. This is even more important for the many older patients who have valve surgery and in whom even a relatively short period of hospitalization can lead to significant functional limitations. ♥

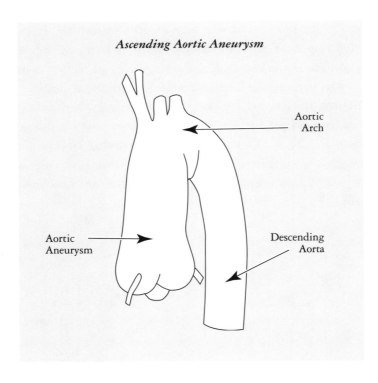

*Ascending Aortic Aneurysm*

Aortic
Arch

Aortic
Aneurysm

Descending
Aorta

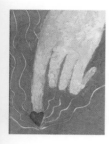

# CHAPTER 12

# Aortic Surgery

*Since the aorta supplies blood* to the entire body, diseases
of the aorta can have important consequences, not the least because
all five liters of the heart's output pass through the aorta every
minute. The two primary diseases that affect the aorta are aneurysm
and dissection.

Aneurysms are areas of weakening of the aortic wall with
consequent enlargement of that segment of the aorta. In some
respects, aneurysms resemble the "bubbles" that used to develop on
bicycle tires. The most common cause of aneurysms is atherosclerosis,
that process of cholesterol plaque build-up that cause coronary artery
disease and heart attack. When this process damages the aortic wall,
narrowing of the large vessel, at least in its components in the chest,
is uncommon. The damage to the aorta, however, can cause weakening
of the wall. This area of weakened wall can thin out and expand,
producing a focal enlargement called an aneurysm.

While atherosclerosis is the most common cause, other conditions less commonly also can produce thoracic aortic aneurysms.
The connective tissues, supporting structures like collagen, which
the body also uses to make scars, are part of the wall of the aorta.
Diseases of connective tissues, like Marfan's syndrome, therefore,
may affect the aorta. The abnormal tissues can also lead to weakening
of the aortic wall and aneurysm formation. Infections of the vessel,
usually in an area of underlying abnormality or trauma to the aorta
are the other most frequent causes. Untreated syphilis, rare today,
used to be a cause of aortic aneurysm. In some patients, there is no
obvious cause.

The natural history of many aneurysms is to enlarge over time. As aneurysms get bigger, they can cause problems just because of their size. When large enough they can push on and compress other cardiac structures or organs in the chest such as the esophagus or the bronchi of the lungs. The most important risk associated with aortic aneurysms, however, is the risk that they will rupture.

Since the aorta is such a large blood vessel, rupture can be catastrophic as it may lead to almost instantaneous loss of a massive amount of blood. Interestingly, however, sometimes the tissues overlying the aorta are sufficiently strong to prevent free rupture. While these contained ruptures require urgent surgical repair, they are not necessarily uniformly fatal. Obviously, though, the primary goal of treatment of aortic aneurysms is to take care of them before they rupture.

Not surprisingly, the risk of rupture of an aortic aneurysm is related both to its absolute size and to its rate of expansion. The normal aorta in the chest has a diameter of about 3 centimeters (cm). When an aortic aneurysm reaches a size of 5.5 cm (nearly twice-normal diameter), most surgeons recommend repair unless the patient has other medical conditions that render a major operation too risky. In patients with connective tissues diseases like Marfan's syndrome, or in those needing heart surgery for other reasons, some surgeons recommend repair of aortic aneurysms even if they do not meet the 5.5 cm size criterion. In some cases like this, repair of 4.5 cm aneurysms is advisable. Alternatively, if an aneurysm enlarges by 0.5 to 1 cm over a six-month period, most surgeons recommend repair since this rapid rate of growth is associated with a higher risk of rupture.

Unruptured aortic aneurysms are often asymptomatic. Sometimes they are first detected when the patient gets a chest X-ray for some other reason and an enlargement consistent with an aortic aneurysm is detected. The definitive diagnosis of both types of thoracic aortic aneurysm can be made with a CT scan or magnetic resonance imaging (MRI) scan. Aortography, an x-ray image obtained by injecting dye into the aorta, was once considered the diagnostic standard but is used much less often now that CT scans and MRI are readily available. It is used today especially to detect involvement of important branches of the aorta (especially the aortic arch vessels) in the aneurysm process.

The surgical approach is to replace the area of aorta involved with the aneurysm. This essentially always involves replacing this segment of the aorta with a synthetic tube graft. Modern grafts are pliable and therefore easier to handle. They are also impregnated with a protein matrix that reduces bleeding. An operation to replace the ascending aorta and/or the aortic arch is done through a standard median sternotomy, an incision down the middle of the breastbone, and with cardiopulmonary bypass. A period of hypothermic circulatory arrest may be used to construct the connection of the graft to the part of the aorta furthest from the heart. This area may involve

*Replacement of Ascending Aorta*

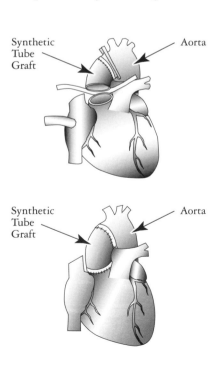

all or part of the aortic arch. Circulatory arrest is necessary to operate in or near the arch of the aorta. It also removes the need to clamp the aorta closed. This may be advantageous when working with a diseased or fragile aorta. When circulatory arrest is used, the patient is placed on the heart-lung machine and the body temperature is reduced to 18-20 degrees Centigrade. The pump can then be turned off and the circulation safely "arrested" for at least thirty minutes — and in some cases, as long as sixty minutes. It is generally better to keep arrest times less than forty-five minutes since the risk of brain injury goes up with longer arrest times. Even in operations for aneurysms which involve the descending thoracic aorta, which are done through an incision in the side of the chest (lateral thoracotomy), bypass and circulatory arrest may be used to avoid clamping the aorta and to protect the spinal cord against injury from lack of blood.

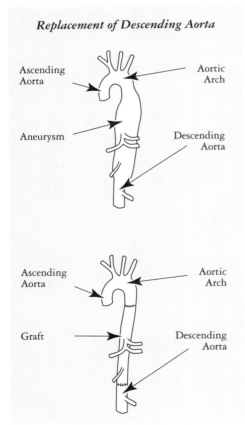

*Replacement of Descending Aorta*

Ascending Aorta

Aortic Arch

Aneurysm

Descending Aorta

Ascending Aorta

Aortic Arch

Graft

Descending Aorta

The ascending aorta is replaced, usually from just above the aortic valve to the inominate artery, the first branch of the aorta in the arch. Similar graft materials are used to replace the descending thoracic aorta. Part, or all of this vessel, may be replaced. Since the blood supply of the spinal cord may be disrupted by replacement of the descending thoracic aorta, many surgeons incorporate inter-costal (between the ribs) branches of the aorta into the repair since these vessels often contribute crucial blood supply to the spinal cord. This reduces the risk of paraplegia (paralysis of the body

### Aortic Dissection

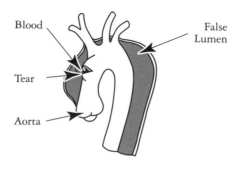

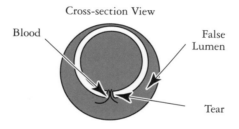

below the waist), one of the most devastating complications of surgery on the descending thoracic aorta.

Dissection, once called dissecting aneurysm, is the most common catastrophe affecting the aorta, more frequent than rupture of an aortic aneurysm. The typical patient is in the seventh or eighth decade of life and has a history of hypertension. Some younger patients with connective tissue disorders such as Marfan's syndrome have increased risk of aortic dissection because of their intrinsic tissue abnormalities.

Dissection begins with a tear in the intima, the inner cellular lining, of the aorta. This loss of intimal integrity allows blood to enter the media (middle muscular layer) of the vessel, where, under the pressure of cardiac contraction, the blood "dissects" along this abnormal tissue plane, creating a "false lumen." This pathological process produces the classic chest or inter-scapular "tearing" pain

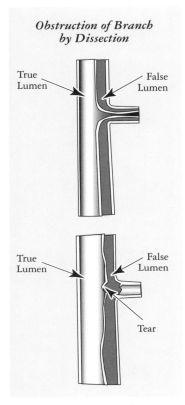

**Obstruction of Branch by Dissection**

True Lumen

False Lumen

True Lumen

False Lumen

Tear

that many patients with this disease describe. As blood dissects the muscular layer of the aorta, critical branches (coronary, carotid, extremity, or mesenteric arteries) can be occluded causing lack of blood flow to the tissues supplied by these vessels. This accounts for the variety of presenting syndromes that aortic dissection can produce. These include heart attack, stroke, injury to abdominal organs, a lack of blood flow to the leg or other parts of the body.

Aortic dissection is a lethal process. Untreated, patients with acute dissection have a mortality rate of 50 percent at twenty-four hours, 75 percent at one week, and 90 percent by one month. The natural history, and therefore the treatment, of aortic dissection are different depending on which parts of the aorta are affected. Dissection involving the ascending aorta, classified as Type A, has different pathological and treatment implications than Type B dissection, which spares the ascending aorta and arch and is confined to the aorta distal to the left subclavian artery.

Many patients with aortic dissection have a history of hypertension and have elevated blood pressure at the time of presentation. Since elevated blood pressure can propagate the dissection process, control of blood pressure and reduction of cardiac contractility constitute the proper initial medical management of nearly all patients with either type aortic dissection. Because the complications of Type A dissection can rapidly be fatal, the definitive treatment of patients with this pathology is nearly always immediate surgery. The operation is designed to prevent the dangerous complications of coronary artery dissection, acute aortic valve insufficiency, or cardiac tamponade (compression of the heart by a blood clot), which can beset patients with Type A dissections.

In Type B dissections, the disease can frequently be managed with blood pressure control alone, unless this therapy fails to control pain, signifying ongoing dissection. The other primary indications for surgery in Type B dissection include compromise of a critical visceral or extremity vessel or aneurysmal dilatation of the false lumen. Under these circumstances, surgery is usually required.

### Type A Dissection

### Type B Dissection

The diagnosis of both types of dissection can usually be made definitively with either transesophageal echocardiography or CT scan. Aortography, once considered the diagnostic standard, is rarely used to detect dissection and, in fact, may miss this diagnosis if there is no flow of dye into the false lumen. Presently, its most important current use is to distinguish whether perfusion of important aortic branches derives from the true or the false lumen. MRI can be used like CT scanning to detect the intimal flap and false lumen of an aortic dissection. This diagnostic test is used less often in part because performance of the procedure requires leaving a potentially unstable patient relatively unmonitored in the powerful magnetic field of the device.

The initial therapy for aortic dissection is to control the dissection process by reducing blood pressure and the propagating force of cardiac contraction. Relief of the patient's pain symptoms determines success. In many instances, the ideal agent to use is esmolol, a short acting, intravenous beta-blocker administered by continuous infusion. This drug lowers blood pressure and helps prevent the reflex increases in heart rate and contractility that often accompany pharmacologic reduction in perfusion pressure. In many patients with Type B dissections confined to the descending thoracic and distal aorta, control of blood pressure, initially with intravenous agents and ultimately with oral anti-hypertensives, constitutes definitive treatment

The treatment of Type A dissection almost always requires an emergency surgical operation. The objectives of this operation are to prevent the previously mentioned potentially fatal complications of involvement of the ascending aorta. These include coronary artery dissection and occlusion, cardiac tamponade, and acute aortic valve insufficiency. It is easy to understand why sudden occlusion of a coronary artery would have dire consequences. Similarly, blood leaking from the false lumen into the pericardium in sufficient volume to produce tamponade would have obvious deleterious effects. The manner in which dissection produces aortic valve dysfunction is less obvious. A competent aortic valve depends on the suspension of the valve cusps by their attachment to the aortic wall. When the proximal aorta is distorted by the false lumen, this suspension is disrupted, causing prolapse of one or more aortic valve leaflets and acute aortic insufficiency. The hemodynamic derangements of acute valve dysfunction are not well tolerated and can produce severe heart failure and intractable cardiogenic shock.

An operation to replace the ascending aorta is the treatment of Type A dissection, which prevents these catastrophic complications. The procedure is done through a standard median sternotomy and with cardiopulmonary bypass. A period of hypothermic circulatory arrest is used to construct the distal anastomosis, which may involve all or part of the aortic arch. Circulatory arrest is necessary to operate in or near the arch. Furthermore and most important, this technique avoids the need to apply a clamp to the fragile dissected aortic tissues. Even in operations for Type B dissections which are done through a lateral thoracotomy, bypass and circulatory arrest are used both to avoid clamping the aorta and for protection of the spinal cord against injury.

The ascending aorta is replaced, usually from just above the aortic valve commissures to the inominate artery. This procedure also resuspends the aortic valve cusps and in most cases, removes the initial intimal tear. It was once the objective of this operation to obliterate the false lumen. Today, however, it is recognized that aortic intimal tears are often multiple (with entry and re-entry points) and that therefore, persistence of a double lumen aorta is common. This is of potential functional importance as frequently critical

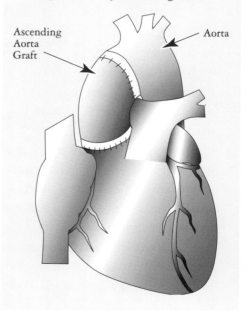

*Replacement of Ascending Aorta*

Ascending Aorta Graft

Aorta

aortic branches are perfused from the false lumen. The development of better graft materials and the use of biological glues have aided hemostasis of the graft and suture lines, once an often-intractable problem. The new woven synthetic grafts are softer, easier to handle and suture, and impregnated with a matrix to improve hemostasis. Biological glues not only act as sealants but also their application toughens the friable aortic tissues improving hemostatic suture placement. Similar considerations apply to replacement of the descending thoracic aorta when that operation is indicated for acute or chronic Type B dissection.

These pharmacologic and technical advances along with improved understanding of the care of the critically ill surgical patient have markedly improved survival and rehabilitation after treatment for aortic dissection. Stroke, paraplegia (for Type B dissection), and multi-system organ failure remain important non-fatal complications but the chance for a patient to survive and recover from this aortic catastrophe has improved especially in the last decade. Early mortality in the modern era is under 10 percent with ten-year long-term survival of 50-65 percent.

The surgical care of patients with aortic aneurysm or dissection requires a co-coordinated approach involving not only the cardio-vascular surgeon and operating room team but also the hospital emergency department, anesthesia, the bypass perfusionists, post-operative nursing and medical consultants. The concerted efforts of these individuals offer hope to patients with major aortic pathologies.

An alternative to surgery is aortic stent grafting, a new procedure, still under investigation, for the treatment of aortic aneurysms and dissections in the chest. Stent grafts are metallic stents, like those placed in coronary arteries, but big enough to work in the aorta and covered with a cloth graft sheath. The cloth graft ensures that the blood flows through the graft after it is in place. As in coronary artery stenting, aortic stent grafts are inserted using catheters rather than during a surgical operation. The stent graft is positioned so that it is anchored above the starting point and below the ending point of the aneurysm or dissection. When deployed, the stent graft excludes the aneurysm or dissection from the circulation as effectively as replacing the same segment of the aorta.

So far, this technology is not perfect. It cannot be used in all locations in the aorta or in all patients. Furthermore, sometimes there are problems with fixation of the graft at the upstream or the downstream end leading to what is called an "endoleak." Endoleaks allow blood into the aneurysmal or dissected aorta, thereby eliminating most of the advantages of the less invasive stent graft approach. Sometimes endoleaks can be fixed by additional catheter procedures but surgery may be necessary. Nonetheless, as stent graft technology is perfected, it is markedly changing the risks of treating major aortic diseases and therefore providing a treatment option for patients who might otherwise not be able to tolerate surgery. ♥

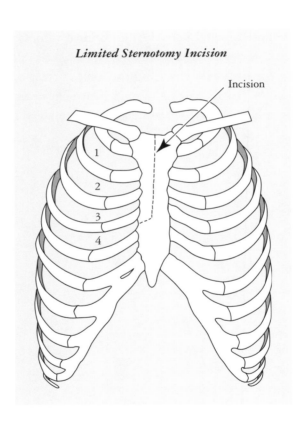

**Limited Sternotomy Incision**

Incision

1
2
3
4

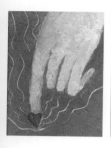

CHAPTER 13

# Minimally Invasive Surgery and Robotics

*Interest in less invasive* or minimally invasive surgical operations has increased in recent years in many specialties, including cardiac surgery. Advances in technology have made several different less invasive approaches possible. In cardiac surgery, minimally invasive has come to mean two things. The first refers to standard operations performed through smaller incisions, with or without videoscopic or even robotic assistance. The second type of less invasive cardiac surgery is off-pump bypass already described in Chapter 9.

Less invasive valve operations on both the aortic and mitral valves can be performed through partial sternotomies or para-sternal (next to the sternum) incisions. The operation is performed in standard fashion under direct vision but the incision is smaller. These smaller incisions have clear-cut cosmetic advantages. In theory, patients may recover faster after an operation done through a smaller incision. This has not been demonstrated convincingly. One report of valve operations done through a partial sternotomy suggests that blood loss and need for blood transfusions may be less than required in a standard operation.

Although advantages beyond a cosmetically pleasing incision have not been proved, there is demand for these procedures from patients and referring doctors. It should be understood, however, that there are potential disadvantages to the small incision approaches. Access to all structures of the heart is limited through a partial sternal incision and some aspects of the standard procedure must be abandoned or done blindly. Flexibility is limited if something unexpected occurs during the operation as well.

Adding video camera assistance and specially designed instruments obviates some of the limitations of the direct vision, small incision approach. Video assisted or video guided operations can be done through ports (very small incisions) and one quite limited "working" incision. A video assisted operation is one done partially under direct vision and partly by visualizing the operative field with a video telescope in the chest. The video images are in two dimensions. Video guided operations are done with all visualization through the video scope. These operations are most applicable to procedures on the mitral valve since they can be done through the right chest. The aortic valve is not accessible through this approach.

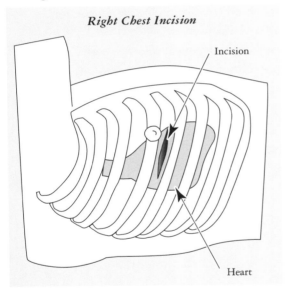

**Right Chest Incision**

Incision

Heart

Such "port access" operations require special cannulas for both the arterial and venous circulations to the heart-lung machine. The arterial cannula incorporates a balloon that is used to exclude blood from the heart and an extra passage for administration of cardioplegia solution. Initial models of this cannula were abandoned since they caused aortic dissection at an unacceptable rate. Current versions seem to have eliminated this problem although balloon migration and rupture remain potential problems. Some surgeons prefer to use a specially designed aortic clamp that is inserted in the chest through a separate small incision and applied externally to the aorta in a standard fashion.

In some centers, these less invasive mitral valve operations are performed through the right chest with the assistance of a surgical robot. There are several versions of such robots currently under evaluation. The most technologically sophisticated incorporates

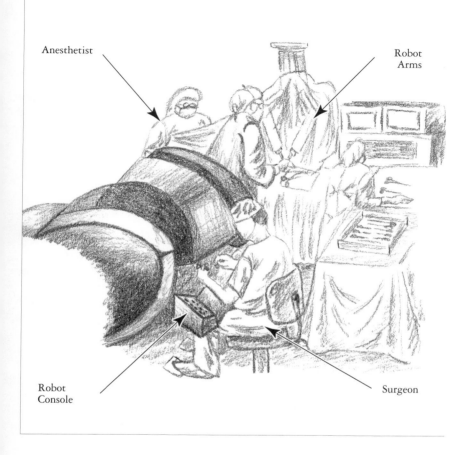

*Surgical Robot*

Anesthetist

Robot Arms

Robot Console

Surgeon

three-dimensional camera visualization and articulating "wrists" that are inserted into the chest. Both technological advances are important.

Three-dimensional visualization obviously provides more natural conditions in which the surgeon can operate. Accurate depth perception is important for accurate placement of incisions and sutures. Even more important is the articulating wrist. This means that motion of the robotic "hands" can be more natural and intuitive for the surgeon. By having the articulating joint inside the chest, there is more flexible movement of the robot arms, especially since the wrist has six degrees of freedom of movement. Current robot technology lacks any kind of tactile feedback. In other words, the surgeon has no sense of how hard or soft a structure may be. Nor does the surgeon have a perception of how much tension is being applied to tissues or sutures. These technological limitations will ultimately be eliminated in the future by microprocessor-controlled versions of surgical robots.

While technologically intriguing, clinical advantages of robotic cardiac surgery have yet to be demonstrated. The operations can be done through smaller incisions, but the procedures take longer and the patient spends more time on the heart-lung machine. Both have the potential to increase side effects and complications. Furthermore, a relatively limited repertoire of operations can be performed with current technology. At present, robotic cardiac surgery is most applicable to operations on the mitral valve and to certain relatively uncommon forms of pathology in the left or right atrium or in the septum between them. The aortic valve is completely inaccessible. Likewise, multi-vessel coronary artery bypass surgery is difficult if not impossible to perform robotically. Nonetheless, this technology is worth investigation by dedicated surgeons who may someday define a new paradigm in cardiac surgery. ♥

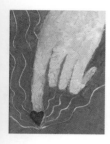

CHAPTER 14

# Heart Failure
# and Heart Transplantation

*In part because of advances* in the medical and surgical
therapy of heart disease, more and more patients are developing
heart failure. This condition is most often due to weakening of the
heart muscle, frequently due to heart attack but sometimes caused
by or associated with problems with the heart valves. Patients with
heart failure are the most rapidly growing group of patients with
heart disease. In the United States, approximately five hundred
thousand patients each year begin treatment for heart failure, and
there are about five million people with this problem.

Replacement of the heart with a normal organ is the most
definitive treatment for heart failure. The first heart transplant was
done in South Africa in December 1967, so heart transplantation is
still in its infancy. Heart transplantation requires a rough size match
between the donor and recipient as well as compatibility matching
for blood type. In the United States donor hearts are apportioned by
region, although inter-regional sharing can occur if a donor organ is
not needed in the region of origin. Priority on the waiting list is
determined by the potential recipient's medical urgency, with sicker
patients having precedence over healthier ones. The other determi-
nant of a recipient's place is the time he or she has spent on the
waiting list.

A heart donor, by definition, is a patient who has died for reasons
other than heart disease. All of these patients have brain death, a
state with rigid clinical criteria. The heart in these patients is still
beating, and therefore, still providing nourishing blood to itself and
all the other organs of the body which, with the exception of the

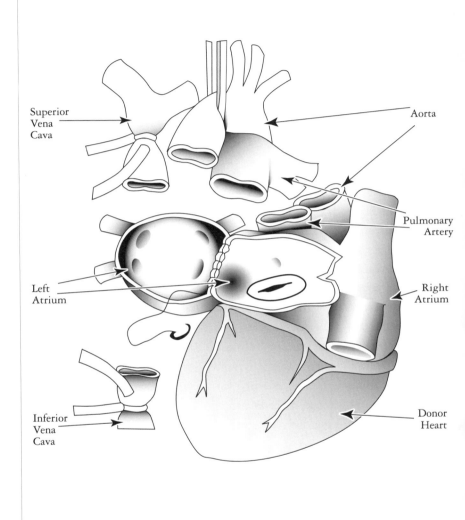

Superior Vena Cava

Aorta

Pulmonary Artery

Left Atrium

Right Atrium

Inferior Vena Cava

Donor Heart

brain, are still living. The donor must be identified and brain death declared by those taking care of the donor patient. The heart transplant team is never involved in the care of donor patients until after brain death has been declared. The whole process of identification of donors and matching the appropriate recipient is handled by an independent regional organ procurement organization.

When a donor organ becomes available, timing of the removal of the donor heart and preparation of the recipient for its implantation is crucial. That is because the maximum safe interval for a heart to be out of the body, and therefore not perfused with blood, is four to six hours. Careful co-ordination of the donor and recipient operations must be planned, particularly since in most situations, multiple organs are harvested from a single donor.

Except in the case of identical twins (a situation that essentially never comes up in heart transplantation) there is never complete tissue matching between donor and recipient. Therefore, all recipients must take powerful medications to prevent their immune systems from identifying the donor organ as foreign, attacking and destroying it. These immunosuppressive medications have important side effects, the most obvious of which is to lower the patient's body defenses, increasing the risk of infection. All recipients, therefore, are poised on a narrow ledge between inadequate immune suppression and rejection of the donor heart—and excessive immune suppression and opportunistic infection. These powerful immunosuppressive drugs also have important non-immunologic side effects. These include high blood pressure, excess body hair growth, neurologic changes, and osteoporosis.

Rejection of a donor heart is determined by pathologic examination of a piece of heart tissue. This heart tissue is obtained by performing a procedure called endomyocardial biopsy. This is done by passing a catheter into a large vein, usually in the neck. A biopsy instrument ("bioptome") is passed through this catheter into the right heart. The small jaws at the end of the bioptome can obtain small pieces of the inside of the right ventricle. Examination of these pieces under a microscopic can reveal the infiltration of immune cells and destruction of heart muscle fibers characteristic of rejection. Most episodes of rejection can be treated by a short period of intensification of the immunosuppressive drugs.

The results of heart transplantation are excellent. One-year survival now exceeds 90 percent, and this is in patients who typically have a one-year survival of less than 50 percent without transplantation. Five-year survival is 70 percent, which is still quite acceptable. Rejection and infection are the primary causes of death early after transplantation. Later, a form of diffuse coronary artery disease peculiar to transplants, and malignancies, which are secondary to the immunosuppressive medications, are the leading causes of death.

Complete replacement of the failing heart is also possible using mechanical devices. These have the advantage of theoretically limitless availability and no need for immunosuppressive drugs. There have been several highly publicized attempts to help patients with heart failure with a total artificial heart. The first of these occurred in the early 1980s and was abandoned because of unacceptable side effects, mainly strokes due to blood clots. The most recent trial of a totally artificial heart is presently ongoing. Unfortunately, this more sophisticated version also appears to be associated so far with an unacceptable rate of blood clots and strokes.

Another potentially promising approach is to use a mechanical device to assist rather than to replace the heart. Several versions of such ventricular assist devices currently are in clinical use. The best are nearly completely implantable, but present versions still require an external power source. In most cases, this requires a wire to traverse the skin. This breach of the skin barrier is a potential source of infection. New technology to allow electrical energy to traverse the skin without a wire may obviate this problem. The other limitation with the implantable devices is that they are restricted to assistance of the left ventricle. In patients who need both right and left heart support, a second device with an external pump must be used to assist the right ventricle.

These limitations aside, ventricular assist devices can be life saving in properly selected patients. They are commonly employed as a "bridge" to transplantation and can help a patient not only survive but be in less critical condition when an appropriate donor organ becomes available. In fact, patients can undergo substantial rehabilitation with these devices. For this reason, left ventricular assist devices (LVADs) are currently under investigation as "destination" therapy for patients with heart failure who are not candidates for transplantation or any other procedure to improve their heart failure.

These devices provide excellent mechanical support of the heart and allow patients to resume nearly normal activity levels. The modern versions are not plagued by blood clots, even with relatively minor levels of anticoagulation. The two primary limitations currently appear to be infection and device failure. With any large, implanted foreign body, infection is a danger especially when a power cable must traverse the skin. Trans-cutaneous energy coils that eliminate breaching the skin with a wire may reduce this latter problem. Unfortunately, mechanical failure of these devices, sometimes catastrophic, has been observed with the current models after longer periods of implantation. While the devices can be repaired or even replaced, this is costly both in terms of patient complications and in economic terms.

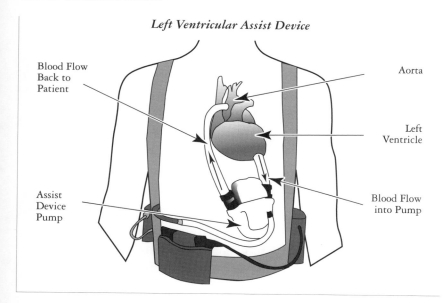

*Left Ventricular Assist Device*

Replacing the failing heart by transplantation from a human donor or replacement with an artificial heart is theoretically attractive. There are close to fifty thousand patients who would benefit from heart replacement. In fact, however, this is not practically possible. First, there are only about two thousand donor hearts available in the United States each year, and because of this shortage, transplantation is only available to relatively few of the sickest patients. While there have been technological improvements in artificial mechanical devices, none is presently perfect and all have persistent problems with blood clots, infection, and the need for external power supplies.

These realities have motivated surgeons to develop other techniques to help patients with heart failure. Unfortunately, many patients and their doctors may not realize that these options exist to improve both the length and the quality of life for some patients with loss of heart function. While medicines can be very helpful, many patients may also be candidates for new surgical procedures to help increase the function of the heart and the quality of the patient's life. These procedures can be divided into procedures that improve the blood supply to the heart, procedures that correct primary or secondary valve problems, especially of the mitral valve, and procedures to remodel the left ventricle, the primary pumping chamber of the heart.

The coronary arteries supply blood to the heart muscle and when they become obstructed by atherosclerosis, they can cause heart attacks. In some patients with diffuse, three-vessel coronary artery obstructions, the heart muscle may lose function but not become permanently damaged. This ischemic, so-called "hibernating" myocardium can be restored to more normal function by improving the blood supply to the heart muscle. In patients with multi-vessel coronary disease, the best way to do this is with coronary artery bypass surgery. In patients with diffuse, ischemic cardiomyopathy in whom it can be demonstrated that the heart muscle is viable, bypass surgery can improve cardiac function, make heart failure disappear, or at least be easier to manage, and significantly improve the patient's quality of life.

Patients with heart failure often have significant dilatation of the heart, especially the left ventricle. This enlargement often stretches the annulus of the mitral valve, leading to significant mitral insufficiency. Alternatively, severe mitral insufficiency can lead to progressive ventricular enlargement and ultimately myocardial failure. In either event, the progressive enlargement increases the insufficiency of the mitral valve, which increases the volume overload of the heart leading to increasing heart failure in an accelerating downward spiral. Somewhat counter-intuitively, mitral valve repair has been shown not only to arrest this continued deterioration, but also to lead to improvements in overall ventricular function. An important component of this response is the preservation of the entire mitral valve apparatus including the chordae and the papillary muscles. Earlier results of mitral valve replacement in heart failure were unfavorable since the conventional way to replace the valve involved resection of the chordal attachments as well as the mitral leaflets. It turns out that the function of the ventricle is as dependent on the normal structure of the mitral valve as the function of the valve is dependent on the normal function of the ventricle. Repairing the former can lead to dramatic improvements in the latter.

Some patients with heart failure after anterior wall myocardial infarction may be candidates for the SAVER (surgical anterior ventricular reconstruction) operation. This surgery, which is usually combined with coronary bypass, remodels the shape of the heart damaged by heart attack so that it functions more efficiently. Studies have confirmed that this operation is beneficial for certain patients with areas of the heart that contract poorly due to previous heart attacks and symptomatic heart failure. The operation changes the shape and size of the left ventricle, improving muscle mechanics and efficiency. These changes also may trigger biochemical remodeling which may enhance the benefits of this procedure further.

Patients with heart failure need not always suffer the limitations cardiac conditions impose, despite partial benefit from medical therapy. All the procedures described — coronary revascularization, mitral valve repair, and surgical ventricular reconstruction —

induce beneficial changes in ventricular shape and function. Heart failure is thought to occur in part through deleterious ventricular remodeling. The concept of beneficial ventricular remodeling may explain the efficacy of surgical procedures that in the past were thought to offer too little benefit and excessive risk in patients with symptomatic heart failure.

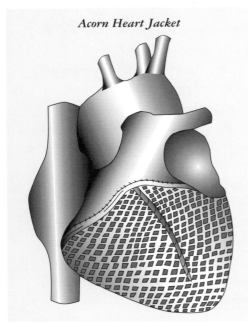

*Acorn Heart Jacket*

Finally, several new devices are under investigation. These share the trait that they change the mechanical or loading conditions of the heart in a presumed effort to induce positive remodeling. Two examples include the Acorn heart jacket and the Myosplint strut. The Acorn jacket is a cloth "sock" that is placed over the ventricles. The sock is not distensible and therefore places a limit on how much the heart can dilate. Preliminary studies suggest that this constriction actually produces beneficial changes in heart function. The Myosplint is a strut device that changes the shape of the heart by constricting it transversely. This essentially helps change the shape of the heart from a dysfunctional spherical form to a more normal and therefore more functional oblong configuration. The long-term efficacies of these and other similar devices remain to be demonstrated. ♥

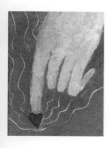

CHAPTER 15

# Women and Heart Disease

*Recent analysis* has shown that heart disease historically has been under-diagnosed and under-treated in women. This gender difference has directly affected the management of coronary artery disease in women. While coronary vascular disease remains the most important public health problem in both women and men, abnormalities of the cardiac valves cause significant disability in affected patients. In both female and male adults, the aortic and mitral valves are most commonly affected. Acquired lesions, by far, out-number congenital anomalies in adults. All of them are amenable to surgical treatment, which is the only therapy that corrects the actual anatomic and functional abnormality. Medical therapy of valvular disease remains palliative and the treatment of choice only in patients in whom the disease is relatively mild or for whom surgery presents unacceptable risk.

The symptoms and signs of coronary artery disease may by atypical in women. Rather than the classic anginal chest pain (pressure, tightness, heaviness), women may experience such non-specific symptoms as nausea, shortness of breath, arm heaviness, or merely a diffuse anxiety. This, coupled with the erroneous assumption that women are "protected" from this form of heart disease has, in the past, led to delays in diagnosis and treatment of women.

Not only has the diagnosis been delayed, but analysis has shown that women have been less likely to receive aggressive management of coronary disease with angioplasty and bypass surgery. One observation is that women do less well after bypass surgery when compared to men. There have been a number of speculations as to the cause of this discrepancy in results. Possible culprits include the fact that, in general, women and their coronary arteries are smaller than those in men — and therefore angioplasty or operations are more difficult to perform on them. Perhaps more plausibly, however, results in women may have been inferior because the diagnosis of coronary disease has been delayed and they have been treated at a more advanced, and therefore higher risk, stage of the disease. Understanding the importance and the specific manifestations of coronary artery disease in women must improve if death and disability are to be reduced.

Education of women and their doctors is crucial for the proper management of this form of heart disease in women.

As noted before, aortic stenosis is the most common lesion of the aortic valve presenting in adults. In younger patients, aortic insufficiency occurs with greater frequency. Both usually require valve replacement since the results of valve repair are unsatisfactory. Mitral insufficiency is by far more common than mitral stenosis in an affluent population where the incidence of rheumatic mitral stenosis is low. In disadvantaged patients, or in those recently immigrated from developing countries, mitral stenosis due to rheumatic fever may present for surgical correction. Interestingly, rheumatic mitral stenosis is more common in women than in men. The first choice operation for either stenosis or insufficiency of the mitral valve is valve repair — although valve replacement may be necessary in a patient whose mitral valve is severely scarred and calcified.

What special considerations apply to the surgical management of valvular heart disease in women? The most important is the relative contra-indication to anticoagulation with coumadin in women of childbearing age. Coumadin is required in any patient with a mechanical valve replacement device. Since the primary advantage of mechanical prostheses is their greater durability compared to tissue valves, especially in younger patients, this type of valve is recommended often in younger women having valve replacement operations. Yet, women desiring to have children should not take coumadin since it can cause birth defects if given during pregnancy.

These realities have led surgeons to strive to repair the valve in any young women with mitral valve disease and to seek alternative tissue valves with greater potential durability in younger female patients with aortic valve lesions. Young women with symptoms and stenotic mitral valves without insufficiency or excessive scarring and calcification of the leaflets, and especially of the subvalvar apparatus, should undergo catheter-based balloon valvuloplasty or open surgical commissurotomy. All young women with significant mitral insufficiency and any symptom or sign of cardiac decompensation should have valve repair. Valve replacement should be reserved for only the most complex lesions that cannot be repaired reliably.

Since aortic valve repair is often not an effective, durable operation, younger women with aortic valve disease should consider aortic valve replacement with the newer stentless, porcine tissue valves. This valve, which is derived from the aortic valve of a pig's heart, retains the native sinuses of Valsalva and therefore does not require a man-made stent for support of the commissures. The lack of the stent reduces obstruction from artificial material, and theoretically allows for more normal valve leaflet motion and valve apparatus flexion during systole and diastole. These hemodynamic and functional advantages may lead to better performance and durability, and thereby provide a tissue replacement device alternative for the younger patient with aortic valve disease requiring replacement but need to avoid long-term anticoagulation with coumadin. ♥

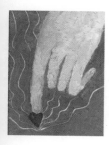

CHAPTER 16

# Athletes and Heart Disease

*Today we are all athletes.* Since heart disease is the most common ailment affecting western societies, we are all athletes with heart disease. What special considerations apply to athletes with heart disease?

Since coronary artery disease is the most common cause of heart disease in adults, how should its management change in patients who desire to remain physically active? While it may seem that the size of the surgical incision might be an important consideration in a patient who wants to resume vigorous physical activity, this is a relatively minor consideration since once even a full sternotomy is healed, it should present no limitation to physical activity.

The most important consideration in the athlete with coronary disease is the need to anticipate a more aggressive use of angioplasty, stent, and coronary artery bypass surgery. The active athlete usually desires to engage in vigorous activity without the threat of heart attack and disabling symptoms. Also, the inconvenience and expense of multiple medications may be undesirable in an individual who wants to be able to participate regularly in sports and games. Therefore, revascularization, either with a catheter or with surgery may be justified in such individuals, even if no survival benefit can be offered.

In patients with valvular heart disease and a desire to engage in exercise programs and sports, earlier intervention for severe valve dysfunction may be indicated. In other words, corrective surgery may be recommended before the patient has either significant symptoms or pathological changes in heart size, shape, or function.

Just as in women of childbearing age, the athlete may desire a valve operation that also avoids the need for coumadin anticoagulation. As in any patient, a durable valve repair operation is the first choice procedure in an athlete as well. When valve repair is not feasible, use of one of the newer tissue prostheses may be indicated. The newer valves have excellent blood flow performance, do not require coumadin, and may have better durability, even in younger patients, than older model tissue prostheses.

Patients interested in athletics should also be interested in prevention of heart disease. Even young healthy individuals who desire to remain active should have a detailed evaluation of cardiac risk factors. Intervention with diet, exercise, and medication programs to modify identifiable risk factors should be done in everyone. The person who embraces the healthy life style of an athlete should be receptive to recommendations for aggressive measures at primary prevention of heart disease.

Even those athlete "weekend warriors" who have developed heart disease should be interested in secondary prevention (modifying risk factors even after development of heart disease). The period after a heart attack, a catheter procedure, or a cardiac operation is a perfect time to capture the attention of a patient who wants to resume an active, physical life. These individuals also should be amenable to formal programs of cardiac rehabilitation that may help them resume their preferred activities sooner.

Athletes — for that matter, everyone — should be motivated to practice all of the components of proper management of heart disease: primary prevention, early diagnosis, aggressive intervention, vigorous rehabilitation, and secondary prevention. These are the supports of a heart healthy life. ♥

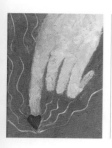

# Conclusion

*This book provides a summary* of modern heart care and heart surgery for the interested patient or potential patient. Since heart disease is so prevalent in our society we are all either patients, potential patients, or related to one or the other. While focusing on the wonderful advances in knowledge, technology, and techniques for the diagnosis and treatment of heart disease, the chapters in this book have also tried to emphasize the importance of a lifetime of management of heart disease.

Heart disease is not something like a cold that you get, you treat, and you cure. Heart disease represents a complex interplay of genetics and modifiable risk factors that require concerted activity by both patients and doctors. Lifetime management, as noted in the last chapter, requires embracing all the components available to doctors and patients. These include early activity in primary prevention, that is, modifying risk factors that can be changed even before heart disease can develop or is detected. When heart disease does occur, it should be aggressively sought-out and diagnosed.

When the disease is identified, its proper management requires careful selection of the variety of medical, catheter, and surgical treatment options available. Disease management does not stop with filling a prescription, a successful angioplasty, or bypass or valve surgery.

Organized cardiac rehabilitation is an important component of disease management that should not be neglected, lest all of the benefits of modern therapy be realized later than necessary, or not at all. Finally, even after the diagnosis and treatment of heart disease, identification and modification of risk factors, secondary prevention, is prudent. It is never too late to minimize the likelihood that this disease, a literal scourge of our society, will progress.

A heart hospital may well be the setting for such modern heart disease management in the near future. Ideally the heart hospital will be built as a "hospital in a hospital" rather than as a freestanding structure off the main hospital campus. The heart hospital in the hospital is preferable since it ensures that patients have access to all the other services provided by a general hospital and which they might need during treatment for their heart condition. In fact, for a variety of reasons, the federal government presently has imposed a moratorium on the construction of freestanding heart hospitals. Nonetheless, the properly designed heart hospital in the hospital of the future will be a center for prevention, diagnosis, treatment, and rehabilitation since it will combine in one readily accessible, logically-organized facility all the services patients require for management of cardiovascular disease.

The heart hospital concept draws on industrial ideas of the "focused factory" which by its defined mission and rational design lead to better, more cost-effective patient care and outcomes. There are increasing numbers of examples of such specialty facilities that are starting to demonstrate both of these advantages. The guiding principles are patient-focused, user-friendly, seamless, and accessible comprehensive care that facilitates lifetime management of cardio-vascular disease.

The concept is to bring services to patients, reduce fragmenta-tion, and to the extent possible, provide a "one-stop" venue for preventative, diagnostic, therapeutic, and rehabilitative cardiovascular services. Implicit in this is a rational facility design that aggregates services in a fashion that mimics how and in what order they are used in the care of patients with cardiovascular disease.

Another advantage of such rational design is the opportunity it affords to build flexibility into service areas. For example, as cardio-vascular technologies evolve, the distinctions between catheterization laboratories and surgical suites will likely diminish; and the ability for "flex usage" of these spaces may become desirable by offering better, more cost-effective care to patients.

Another potential advantage of the heart hospital is the opportunity it may afford to develop new therapies. The frequent interactions of patients and their multiple caregivers may be a fruitful environment that will help stimulate the development of tomorrow's heart care.

These exciting possibilities will provide ideal venues for the heart therapies of today and those of the future that are yet to be conceived. Since heart disease is such an important problem, its management should be of equal importance and interest to us all. This book has been written to help readers understand both the accomplishments and the limitations of the practice of the care of heart disease. To the extent that it contributes to the heart health of us all, its writing will have been a success. ♥

℞

# Prescription for a Healthy Heart

1. Exercise regularly.
2. Eat a balanced diet with reasonable portion sizes.
3. Keep body mass index as close to 25 as possible.
   (Weight in pounds x 704.5/height in inches$^2$)
4. Don't smoke.
5. Don't smoke.
6. Check blood pressure regularly per your doctor and maintain an optimal level.
   (normal 120-140/80)
7. If you have diabetes (high blood sugar) use diet, exercise, weight control, and perhaps medication, to keep blood sugar within desired range.
   (100-150)
8. Have cholesterol (including different types) checked and control different levels with diet, exercise, and medication as directed by your doctor.
9. See your doctor regularly to discuss management of all risk factors (as well as the care and treatment of any other condition you may have).

At the CardioVascular Center at The Chester County Hospital, our philosophy of care focuses on patients and incorporates a new paradigm in the treatment of cardiovascular disease. Our goal is the prevention and treatment of heart disease as the patient experiences it.

We seek to assist our patients and their referring physicians in the continuum of cardiovascular care from primary prevention to early diagnosis, timely intervention, aggressive rehabilitation, and secondary prevention. Our goal is to become a resource for doctors and patients by providing a multi-disciplinary approach to a lifetime of disease management.

The organizing principle of the CardioVascular Center is to offer services that are personalized, integrated, streamlined, and seamless, without arbitrary differentiation between medicine and surgery, inpatient and outpatient, and prevention, diagnosis and treatment. We strive to offer patients and their doctors a congenial atmosphere and easy access to this full spectrum of services for the management of cardiovascular disease.

Finally, the CardioVascular Center is a locus for the advancement of knowledge and for education about cardiovascular disease for doctors and patients. By participating in clinical studies and partnering with national and international leaders in the prevention, diagnosis, and treatment of heart disease, the Center brings the expertise of nationally recognized cardiologists, cardiovascular surgeons, and other health professionals to the care of its patients. ♥

# INDEX

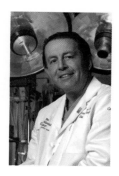

*Dr. Verdi J. DiSesa* is Chief of Cardiac Surgery of the CardioVascular Center at The Chester County Hospital. He received his education at Harvard University and the School of Medicine of the University of Pennsylvania. In his career he has served on the faculties of Harvard Medical School, the University of Pennsylvania, and Rush Medical College. In addition to his outstanding clinical work in heart surgery, Dr. DiSesa is an internationally-recognized teacher, lecturer, and investigator and a member of prestigious national and international organizations dedicated to the diagnosis and treatment of heart disease. He lectures widely about surgical and other therapies for patients with heart problems. Dr. DiSesa lives in Wynnewood, Pennsylvania with his wife and four sons. ♥